PENGUIN BOOKS
PREMEDITATED MAN

Richard M. Restak was graduated from Georgetown University Medical School in 1966. He held psychiatric residencies at Mount Sinai Hospital in New York and a neurology residency at George Washington Hospital and now lives in Washington, D.C., where he practices neurology and neuropsychiatry. Articles by him have appeared in the *Saturday Review, The New York Times,* and the *Washington Post,* and he has served as a consultant for the *Encyclopedia of Bioethics.*

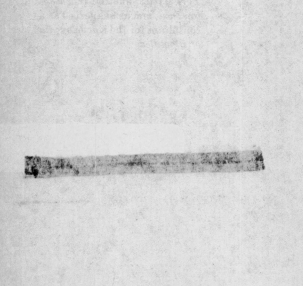

pre-
meditated
man

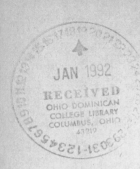

RICHARD M. RESTAK

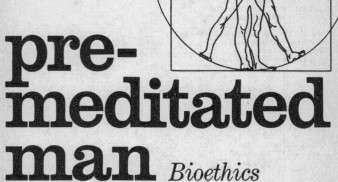

pre-
meditated
man

*Bioethics
and the Control
of Future
Human Life*

PENGUIN BOOKS

Penguin Books Ltd, Harmondsworth,
Middlesex, England
Penguin Books, 625 Madison Avenue,
New York, New York 10022, U.S.A.
Penguin Books Australia Ltd, Ringwood,
Victoria, Australia
Penguin Books Canada Ltd, 2801 John Street,
Markham, Ontario, Canada L3R 1B4
Penguin Books (N.Z.) Ltd, 182–190 Wairau Road,
Auckland 10, New Zealand

First published in the United States of America
by The Viking Press, Inc., 1975
Published in Penguin Books 1977

Library of Congress Cataloging in Publication Data
Restak, Richard M. 1942—
Premeditated man.
Includes index.
1. Bioethics. 2. Medical ethics. I. Title.
QH332.R47 1977 174'.2 76-56358
ISBN 0 14 00.4411 6 (pbk.)

Printed in the United States of America by
Offset Paperback Mfrs., Inc.,
Dallas, Pennsylvania
Set in Linotype Century Expanded

To my mother and father,
and to my wife, Carolyn

Acknowledgments

Those who were personally of great help to me while I researched this book include:

David Allen, Harvard University; George Annas, Boston University School of Law; Bernard Barber, Columbia University; Sarah Broad of the Thalidomide Shareholder's Action Committee, London; Diane Bauer, Children's Defense Fund, Washington, D.C.

Also Donald Chalkley, Institutional Relations Branch of the National Institutes of Health; Guido Calabresi, Yale University Law School; Daniel Callahan, Institute of Society, Ethics, and the Life Sciences, Hastings-on-Hudson, New York.

Also Cedric Carter, Institute for Child Health, London; Alexander Capron, University of Pennsylvania Law School; Steven Chorover, Massachusetts Institute of Technology; William Claiborne, *The Washington Post;* Harold Cohen, Institute for Behavioral Research, Silver Spring, Maryland; Noel Epstein, *The Washington Post.*

Also Murray Falconer, Maudesley Hospital, London; Gary Flamm, National Cancer Institute; John Fletcher, Interfaith, Washington, D.C., and Institute of Society, Ethics, and the Life Sciences; Karl Frank, Laboratory for Neural Control, National Institutes of Neurological Diseases and Stroke; Mark Frankel, Department of Political Science, Wayne State University.

Also, Dorothy Glancy, Staff Council, Subcommittee on Constitutional Rights; Robert Heath, Tulane University School of Medicine; Franz Ingelfinger, *The New England Journal of Medicine.*

Also, Leon Kass, St. John's College, Annapolis, Maryland, and the Kennedy Center for the Study of Human Reproduction and Bioethics; Jay Katz, Yale University Law School; Marc Lappe, Institute of Society, Ethics, and the Life Sciences; Joseph Klutz, research assistant to the House Subcommittee on Constitutional Rights; Christopher Macy, *New Humanist,* London.

Also, Ann McLaren, University of Edinburgh; Joel Meister; Barbara Milstein, The National Prison Project of the American Civil Liberties Union; Robert Neville, Manhattanville College; Lesley Olsner, *The New York Times*.

Also Adrian Peracchio, Yerkes Primate Center, Emory University, Atlanta, Georgia; Elaine Potter, *The Sunday Times*, London; Jerome K. Ravetz, Council for Science and Society, London; Albert Rosenfeld, *Saturday Review;* Paul Sieghart, London; Jack Singer, Guy's Hospital, London; Warren Reich, Kennedy Center for Human Reproduction and Bioethics, Washington, D.C.; Steven Rose, Open University, London.

Also David Sharp, George Washington University Law School; Ted Shotter, London Medical Group, London; Donald L. Snyder, Yale University School of Medicine; Patrick C. Steptoe, Oldham General Hospital, Manchester, England.

Also Anthony Storr, London; Tim Shallice, Maudesley Hospital, London; Anthony Thorley, Reigate, Surrey, England; Robert Veatch, Institute of Society, Ethics, and the Life Sciences; Patrick Wall, University College, London.

Thanks are due specifically to staff and members of the Institute of Society, Ethics, and the Life Sciences in Hastings-on-Hudson, New York, and the Kennedy Center for Human Reproduction and Bioethics in Washington, D.C. Both institutions made their extensive resources available to me, and many of the members of both were extremely generous with their time.

Thanks are due to my wife, Carolyn, for her help and inspiration; and to my editor, Elisabeth Sifton of The Viking Press, whose suggestions have been invaluable throughout the writing of the book.

Finally, special thanks to David Obst, agent and friend.

R.M.R.

Martha's Vineyard, 1974
Washington, D.C., 1975

Contents

Introduction: What Bioethics Is About

Within the next ten years we are going to witness a social revolution quite unlike anything we have seen before: a revolution in our ways of thinking about our minds and our bodies. The nature of the forces operating to bring about this change will be strikingly different from what we usually associate with social revolutions. In this instance biomedical technology rather than predominantly political issues will be the stimulus for social change.

The cures for now fatal diseases, along with their earlier detection; an understanding and retardation of the processes of aging; new techniques to control the behavior of vast numbers of people; the harnessing of more bacteria and viruses to produce new chemicals and foods—some of these are already possible, and others will be in the foreseeable future. It's all part of an explosion of biomedical expertise, an explosion that is creating many critical issues: How can we reap the benefits of biomedical technology without letting it destroy us? How can we prevent the erosion of valuable human qualities it has taken us thousands of years to achieve?

Only recently has a scientific specialty emerged concerned with questions such as these. It is known as bioethics, and it seeks answers to questions as varied as: Is psychosurgery a legitimate method of psychiatric treatment? Should there be rules governing human experimentation? This book is a response to such questions.

Some years ago I set myself the goal of finding out at first hand what biomedical advances were reasonably likely to be made in the next decade, as well as to anticipate their probable effect on our lives. To do this I enlisted the aid of many of the scientists and bioethicists who studied and wrote on these subjects. In every possible instance I met with them and discussed their perceptions of where we're headed. I wasn't long at this task, however, before I realized that things were even more complex than I had imagined.

The first and most difficult problem was to find the framework that encompassed such superficially unrelated issues as cloning, psychosurgery, and sperm banking. As I proceeded there were times when none of these seemed to fit together. I seemed to be dealing with dozens of related issues, but what exactly did they have in common? What did genetic engineering, for instance, have to do with behavior-modification programs used in the prisons? One obvious answer was that biomedical technology had made each of these things possible. This was one approach. But it seemed like concentrating on the props and the costuming at the expense of the play.

Unfortunately many of my conversations with the people concerned with these matters were not very helpful in this regard. A person who studies the effects of sex predetermination on family structure could not care less about psychosurgery. Another, laboring over detailed guidelines for human experimentation, did not consider computer health data banks as a problem. In a word, things seemed chaotic.

After several hundred hours of interviews I began to get a "handle" on the issues that enabled me to pull them all together into a system that made sense for me. Let me try briefly to explain what I mean.

As with many other questions in a free society, questions regarding the human consequences of biomedical technology involve questions of power. Should a scientist have the power to conduct experiments that may be harmful to the experimental subjects? Should a parent have the power to determine the genetic characteristics of a child? Should the government have the power to control the behavior of its citizens? Looked at from this vantage point the questions are, I believe, manageable. Instead of searching for absolute answers to absolute questions like "What is ethical?" or "What is good?" by concentrating instead on practical issues of power, we can arrive at workable solutions. What is allowable? How can we achieve the greatest good for the greatest number while still protecting the rights of minorities? These are essential questions that we *can* try to answer. To me they form the basis for the elucidation of a meaningful bioethics.

Many may disagree with me that questions of right

and wrong, ethical and unethical, may be put to one side in the formulation of a bioethics. They may be right, and I respect their opinion; but so far no one has formulated how *in vitro* fertilization, for instance, can be evaluated strictly in terms of its ethicality. Is it ethical or unethical to help a sterile woman to have a child by means of fertilization outside her womb? And what is the ethics of widespread laboratory reproduction completely divorced from human sexuality? When viewed in terms of pure ethics these questions become incapable of resolution, it seems to me, and no more meaningful than the medieval theologians' debate over how many angels dance on the head of a pin. A much more useful approach is to judge such biomedical techniques as *in vitro* fertilization in the context of the question how much power one group—scientists—should be allowed to exert over our lives. Viewed in this way, bioethics is concerned with defining the allowable limits of scientific power.

During the last several years there have been indications that some scientists at least envision no limitations on their power. As one of them told me, speaking of laboratory methods of human reproduction, "The scientifically possible must become our mandate. What can be done must be done." Such scientific elitism should come as no surprise. Far and away the largest single sponsor of biomedical research in the United States today is the government. That is supposed to mean us, *you and me*. Yet I don't ever remember hearing a public discussion on whether or not public funds should be made available for the heart-transplant programs that have already fallen into disuse. Who decided that kidney machines should be developed to treat incurable kidney disease, with the result that thousands of patients are condemned to die because somebody cut off those funds before enough machines and personnel became available? Who decides which of those patients will be selected for the renal-dialysis program? They are not questions of "ethics," they are questions of power. So far, few people have questioned whether scientists should have this kind of power.

Intimately linked with biomedical technology are not only our health but the length and the quality of our lives.

There can be no turning back from that dependence. We are beyond that now. Biotechnology is here, a given; it must somehow be adjusted to and, in future, anticipated. Even to ignore its consequences is to decide by default the controversies it creates and the decisions it demands. For key decisions will be made within the next two or three years; they cannot be avoided. Like it or not, we are going to have to come to grips with such issues as whether we should pass laws to have compulsory tests for certain hereditary diseases or whether we should engineer genetic changes that seem to us desirable in our children.

Understandably, most of us haven't given much thought to such matters. In the past, scientific advances proceeded at a rate consistent with our response times for adjustment. We have had almost two generations to adapt to the automobile, for instance; now our poisoned environment is forcing us to think again about the overall effects of the internal combustion engine on the quality of our lives. The jet plane and nuclear fission were invented only a generation ago; antibiotics have been used for only half a generation, tranquilizers and antidepressant drugs less than twenty-five years, organ transplantation less than ten. The response time—in which we can anticipate and plan for the consequences of the changes likely to result from biotechnology—is becoming shorter and shorter. It is impossible for any one of us to think out all the probable implications of promised biotechnical advances.

This increasingly shortened response time, combined with more dreadful consequences of error, are forcing us to reach decisions more quickly, and most important, to get them right *the first time around*. We can no longer proceed in the time-honored tradition of "waiting and seeing" the results of biomedical advances. Today, the premature introduction of an incompletely tested drug may quickly result in the birth of thousands of deformed children. Or the destructive effect of a new drug may, like a time bomb, occur years after its introduction. Some of the complications arising from the taking of oral contraceptive pills, for instance, were documented only several years after their worldwide distribution. For two of my own patients, women helplessly paralyzed and speechless at the ages of nineteen and twenty-eight as a result of strokes brought on by birth-control pills, the biotechnology leading to the development of oral contraception was clearly not a happy one. Our response time has caught up with us: we must consider the likely consequences of a new biotechnique *simultaneously* with its introduction.

Let me take up one objection before proceeding further. There is a claim that most people do not care and cannot be made to care about the human consequences of biomedical technology. A variant of this is the claim that the issues are too specialized for the general public. These views are contradicted by many recent experiences. Without going into the wisdom of the Supreme Court's most recent decision on abortion, we can say that the public debate about abortion showed once and for all that issues regarding the human application of biomedical technology really do engage the interest, even the passions, of large numbers of people. Unrestricted abortion still remains a topic likely to generate more heat than enlightenment in open discussion.

The thalidomide tragedy in England provides another recent example. In response to a brilliant series of articles in the *Sunday Times* of London, some of the shareholders of National Distillers Inc., which developed and marketed thalidomide in England, united into a shareholders' action group for the purpose of forcing the company to pay a just settlement to these children. While in London researching this book, I spent several days with members of the group and personally witnessed a most extraordinary commitment and concern in the interest of justice for more than three hundred children whose lives had been wrecked by biotechnology. In a very real sense the members of the action group are, as stockholders in Distillers, meting out their own money, having engaged in tremendously complicated, expensive, and frustrating negotiations with their board of directors. Due to the combined efforts of the *Sunday Times* and the shareholders, a hope now exists for an eventual resolution of the legal impasse that has existed since 1962. People do care and care passionately about the human consequences of biomedical technology.

Now for an overview of what this book is about.

Part One, "Psychosurgery and the Cult of Behavior Control," grew out of my interest as a neurologist in the gadgetry now being used to modify people's behavior. Psychosurgery is, of course, the most dramatic form of behavior-control technology now in use. But I am concerned now less with the gadgetry than I am with the larger question of the appropriateness of behavior-control technology in a free society. From my study of psychosurgery I became interested in other, more pernicious, forms of behavior control. I discovered that in the last four years our government has invested large sums in the development of behavior-modification "treatment" programs in American prisons and mental hospitals—all of it accomplished, incidentally, without any of the cross-disciplinary evaluations that usually precede the commitment of public funds to behavior or social science research. Already these programs have been set up to "control" the behavior of some of the most inarticulate and helpless members of our society. At the conclusion of this section I discuss how this came about, and why it must be stopped.

Part Two, "Genetic Engineering: Opportunity or Trap?" examines the most publicized aspect of the new genetic engineering: *in vitro* fertilization, the "test-tube baby" controversy. It also deals with a subject of even more immediate concern: the rapidly expanding practice of anonymous sperm donation and the profound effects it will have on our traditional belief in genetic identity. I let a world-famous obstetrician tell us what he thinks about the whole notion of "preselection" for physical and mental traits, and I explore the elements in a very sophisticated genetic-counseling unit at Guy's Hospital in London. Experience both in England and in America shows that hastily drawn proposals based on faulty or mistaken genetic propositions can lead to social disaster. In "What Price the Perfect Baby?" I tell the story of one man's research on the effect that the new genetic engineering is already having on our attitudes toward what constitutes meaningful human life.

In Part Three, "The Animal of Necessity," I explore the problems raised by human experimentation. In 1972 national recognition was given to a study sponsored by the government which for decades had drafted large numbers of unwitting and uninformed men into a long-term study of syphilis. This was a supposedly rare and unprecedented bio-medical catastrophe. But alarming experiments on human beings are in fact not rare at all and constitute a medical tradition that can be traced back at least two hundred years. As a rule these experiments do not come to public attention but remain safely camouflaged by scientific jargon and the patter of statistics. Every so often, however, something like Tuskegee erupts into a public outrage—but then it is soon forgotten, and all too soon the experimenters are back to business as usual.

Next, I turn attention to the people engaged in human experimentation. Our preconceptions about the ethical characteristics of medical researchers contrast starkly with what they're really like as revealed by an in-depth study by a sociologist at Columbia University.

One idea that seems to offer some hope that we can arrive at a definition of what is allowable in human experimentation is the notion of "informed consent": the process by which a research subject voluntarily agrees to participate in an experiment, after the dangers and side effects have been fully explained to him. Actually, informed consent is a lot more difficult than it first appears and, in some instances, is impossible to achieve. I discuss these situations and why certain ongoing experiments must be stopped.

In the last two years, radically different experiments have been devised that tell us amazing things about our bodies and our minds. Soon we'll be light-years away from our present simplistic vision of someone in a white lab coat administering a new drug to evaluate its usefulness. In the section entitled "The Opening Wedge" I present portions of conversations I have had with a bioethicist named Dr. Marc Lappe, who explains how these new experiments will challenge "our concept of our own humanity." I also discuss the reasons why "medical" experiments constitute only a small part of present human experimentation. Some of the most alarming experiments are secretly taking place in settings as unlikely as public rest rooms or the barracks of military installations. It's all part of the research method of a new group of experimentalists to whom nothing is sacred.

"The Search for Solutions" explores the options available to us for making certain something like the Tuskegee study never happens again. One of them, H.R.7724 (popularly known as the Kennedy bill), has passed into law; the other, a proposal for a National Human Investigation Board, remains only another piece of paper on the desk of the Surgeon General. A much more promising approach is the brainchild of a concerned group in England, The Council for Science and Society, and I discuss why I think they might come up with the answers we need.

Lastly, I have tried to come to some tentative conclusions about how we can humanize biotechnology. Here I've attempted to integrate my experiences as a physician, writer, scientist, and concerned citizen. Certainly the questions we must answer about biomedical technology are not easy questions. They may ultimately turn out to be unanswerable, and what seems desirable today may be inappropriate tomorrow. People change, our society changes; how then can we expect that our earliest gropings toward a bioethics will be anything but provisional? But this doesn't absolve us from the obligation to try. In the long run bioethics may turn out to be the most important body of knowledge we have ever attempted to define.

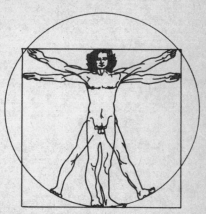

Part One

Psychosurgery and the Cult of Behavior Control

Of Chimpanzees,
Ice Picks,
and Madmen

Dr. Orlando J. Andy is every inch a Southern gentleman. Quiet spoken, impeccably dressed, now in his mid-fifties, Dr. Andy would fit right into the role of a plantation-owner in an updated version of *Gone With the Wind*. Behind his gentility and ingratiating manner, however, lies a single-minded dedication to a cause: the control of violently aggressive behavior. After thirteen years as chairman of the Department of Neurosurgery at the University of Mississippi School of Medicine in Jackson, Dr. Andy is today one of America's leading proponents of psychosurgery as a solution to chronic psychiatric disease.

Dr. Andy has made his position very clear; at a conference on psychosurgery sponsored by the National Institute of Mental Health he had this to say: "All abnormal behavior results from structurally abnormal brain tissue. Psychiatric techniques are now in most instances futile in dealing with these abnormalities. In fact, adequate therapy can be obtained only by techniques, such as surgery, which deal directly with the structurally abnormal brain tissue." When pressed on this point, however, Dr. Andy admitted that no one has demonstrated abnormalities in the structural brain tissue in psychiatric disease. Still, he continued, "It is unfortunate that our institutions are constantly filled with patients having behavioral disorders which do not respond to psychiatric and medical therapy and which would respond to surgery but are denied appropriate treatment for a variety of rational and irrational reasons. My own clinical interest has been in the realm of controlling aggressive, uncontrollable, violent, and hyperactive behavior which does not respond to medical or psychiatric therapy. I have developed a clinical description of such behavior: THE HYPERRESPONSIVE SYNDROME. This is erratic, aggressive, hyperactive, and emotional instability which in its most full-blown expression terminates in attack. These are the patients who need surgical treatment. In addition, there are others: Patients who are a detriment to themselves and society; custodial patients who require constant attention, supervision, and an inordinate amount of institutional care. It should be used in children and adolescents in order to allow their developing brain to mature with as normal a reaction to its environment as possible."

Dr. Andy went on to explain that many of his subjects have been children aged seven and over; one was a child of five. The goal in each case was "to reduce the hyperactivity to the levels manageable by parents." Dr. Andy has performed between forty and fifty operations—he's not sure exactly how many. Several children have had more than one operation; in at least one case, five operations were required to bring about "behavioral control."

At one point during Dr. Andy's address, he was interrupted by a question regarding the medical ethics of his psychosurgical procedures. He replied: "The ethics involved in the treatment of behavioral disorders is no different from the ethics involved in the treatment of all medical disorders. The medical problems involving behavior have a more direct impact on society than other medical problems such as coronary or kidney disease. Still, if treatment is desired, it is neither the moral nor the legal responsibility of society to decide what type of treatment should be administered. The ethics for the diagnosis and treatment of behavioral illness should remain in the hands of the treating physician."

This idea of modifying behavior by surgically cutting parts of the brain is not new. First references to such a procedure can be traced to Roman times when it was observed that insanity might be relieved by a sword wound to the head. But all modern psychosurgical methods date from the physiologist James Fulton's observation in 1935 that when he cut a specialized group of nerve fibers from the frontal lobes of the brains of two chimpanzees, Becky and Lucy, it was possible to tame the animals. After the operation, the chimps could remember old tricks, even learn new ones, but they accepted test situations and frustrations with "philosophical calm." That same year Egas Moniz, a Portuguese neurologist, attended the International Congress of Neurology in London and heard Fulton report on his chimps' postoperative changes in behavior. Moniz asked, "If frontal lobe surgery prevents the development of neurosis in animals, why would it not be feasible to relieve anxiety states in people by means of surgery?" Fulton wrote years later in his memoirs that he was "shocked" by the suggestion that the technique be applied to humans. But the very next year, Dr. Moniz persuaded his neurosurgical colleague Almeida Lima to perform the first "psychosurgical" operation in a mental hospital in Lisbon. The patient, a sixty-three-year-old woman diagnosed as a severe depressive, was released as cured two months after her operation. Nineteen more patients underwent similar operations as Dr. Moniz set in motion his plan "to modify the mental life of some lunatics by destroying parts of the frontal lobes." Thirteen years later Moniz won the Nobel prize in medicine and was commended for "the development of prefrontal leucotomy in the treatment of certain psychoses." The number of lobotomies, as this procedure came to be called, performed by Dr. Moniz is unknown. He retired early from his neurologic practice, several years before a violent death at the hands of a crazed former patient.

In 1942 Walter Freeman, a neurologist, and James Watts, a neurosurgeon, both at George Washington University Hospital in Washington, D.C., reported that extreme depression and agitation—even hallucinations—could be greatly alleviated by cutting the fibers leading from the frontal lobe of the brain to the neighboring thalamus. The connections between these two structures are normally responsible for a delicate interplay between thought (a frontal-lobe function) and emotion (at least partly a thalamic function). After cutting these connections, the doctors reported that exaggerated emotional responses decreased. Although hallucinations might continue, they would be far less terrifying.

The Freeman-Watts treatment spread quickly, and during the 1940s somewhere in the range of fifty thousand patients were lobotomized in the United States alone. Dr. Freeman was a lobotomy zealot and calculated that he had personally performed more than 3500 operations, using a gold-plated icepick which he carried with him in a velvet-lined case. After the local application of a mild pain-killer, Dr. Freeman would plunge the icepick through the thin bone of the upper inner angle of the eye socket, severing the frontal nerve connections to the thalamus. No elaborate preparations or precautions preceded this grisly operation, which often took place in the patient's home or in Dr. Freeman's office at St. Elizabeths Hospital. Dr. Freeman's enthusiasm for "ice pick surgery" knew no bounds; several former associates can recall long lines of patients waiting for treatment outside his office.

Unfortunately, these lobotomies, especially as practiced by Dr. Freeman, often resulted in the zombielike state known as the "frontal lobe syndrome." Common symptoms included indifference to other people, convulsive seizures, and intellectual impairment. Patients often became self-centered and utterly dependent on others for the simplest routines of day-to-day living.

Since that time, psychosurgeons have developed a less crude method of eliminating undesired emotional responses. The procedure involves tampering with what has come to be known as the limbic system. Stated at its simplest, the "limbic system" includes the structures of the limbic lobe along with all the other brain structures with which there are established connections.* In 1937 Dr. J. Papez of the University of Chicago postulated the existence of a network of nerve-cell connections that produced "a harmonious mechanism which may elaborate the functions of central emotion, as well as participate in emotional expression." Dr. Papez, although certainly not ignoring the role of the frontal lobes in emotional expression, chose instead to concentrate on a rim of brain tissue forming the medial border (limbus) of the cerebral hemispheres. In a classic paper entitled "A Proposed Mechanism of Emotion," Dr. Papez demonstrated the importance of subcortical structures in emotion. In lower animals these structures form the basis for emotional reactions. Tampering with the amygdala in an animal, for instance, produces drowsiness, in-

---

* The limbic system, although still not totally defined, includes the subcallocal, cingulate, fornicate, and parahippocampal gyri, as well as the underlying hippocampal formation dentate gyrus and that cortico medial part of the amygdaloid.

difference to surroundings, loss of appetite, and a peculiar symptom known as psychic blindness. The animal may stare for hours at food, not realizing that it is meant to be eaten. Studies on the human limbic system have established the existence of emotional centers similar in structure and presumably in function to those found in lower animals. Proponents of operations on these limbic areas argue that they produce less "blunting" of the personality than is caused by operations involving the frontal lobes.

But recent work has invalidated any strict separation of the frontal lobes in the limbic system. And indeed, the two-way connections between the medial portions of the frontal lobe and the limbic system suggest, in the words of one researcher, "the frontal cortex both monitors and modulates the limbic mechanisms." Thus, after thirty-five years of research we are arriving at a more unified concept of brain function as it relates to behavior.

Although it is fairly simple to describe the general organization of the limbic system, its finer details are very complex. For example, the preoptic area of the rat has an extremely tiny, intricate organizational structure comprising five different regions. These, in turn, occupy only one-twentieth of the volume of the preoptic area. Thus, even the smallest lesion, however skillfully placed, would destroy other structures, many with presently unknown functional properties. And the preoptic area is only one component of the limbic system; almost any lesion made in other portions of the system would have the same potential for destroying large numbers of unrelated and perhaps critically important structures. Applying this type of experimental data to psychosurgery emphasizes our present uncertainties; in the current state of the art no one can guarantee that a psychosurgical procedure done by any surgeon, no matter how skilled, will result in exactly the effect desired and no other. This should be contrasted with more routine surgical procedures such as an appendectomy where, barring unforeseen complications, fairly precise predictions of result can be made.

With the discovery of tranquilizers in the early 1950s, interest in surgery on both the frontal lobes and limbic system declined sharply. A drug called Thorazine was widely used as a kind of chemical lobotomy. Agitated and hallucinating patients became calm and manageable under the influence of the new chemical, without suffering the permanent blunting effect of lobotomies. It soon was apparent, however, that the use of this miracle drug carried its own penalties, particularly drug allergies, serious blood abnormalities, paradoxical reactions resulting in further excitement rather than calm, and a bizarre disorder of muscle tone and movement known as tardive dyskinesia. These failures resulted in a resurgence of interest in psychosurgery.

In the last twenty years, at least eight different surgical procedures have been developed in which surgical incisions are made in one or more portions of the limbic system. The two most common operations used today are cingulotomies and amygdalotomies, which involve deep cuts in these two key areas of the emotional brain. According to limbic-system theory, disturbed emotional patterns (e.g., violence, deep depression, suicidal tendencies) are in part the result of a form of "short circuitry" between the limbic system and the rest of the brain. Cutting the amygdala or cingulum is intended to interrupt these faulty "connections" in the hope that new "connections" will develop and that the interruption will abolish the disturbed behavior patterns. In actuality the correlation between behavior and limbic structures is at best disputable.

Surgical advances in the last fifteen years have led to increasingly precise "targets" within the limbic system. The most innovative development involves a special type of psychosurgical procedure developed in response to the need for pinpoint accuracy, within millimeters, as well as three-dimensional visualization. The method known as stereotactic surgery allows the predetermination of the site of surgical incision in relation to easily recognizable anatomical landmarks. To do this, the patient's head is first shaved and then placed in an open geometric frame which is rigidly attached to the skull by drillpoints that penetrate into the outer table of bone. When the frame is positioned, air is introduced into the inner cavities of the brain: the ventricles. "Target zones" for lesion making are then plotted on a three-dimensional grid in relation to parts of the air-outlined ventricular system. Through tiny burr holes an externally guided probe is introduced, enabling three-dimensional visualization and the placing of tiny "lesions" in selected parts of the brain.

One of the first uses of stereotaxis was in relieving Parkinson's disease, a neurologic disorder marked by slowness of movement and tremors. Neuroanatomical data, accumulated from animal experiments, pointed to the brain's caudate nucleus as important in Parkinsonian tremor. A small, deeply situated brain site, the caudate nucleus did not lend itself to the comparatively crude neurosurgical methods in use during the pre-stereotactic era. With stereotaxis, however, the caudate can be visualized and "lesioned" with often stunning results. Such operations became less frequent with the introduction of the replacement drug L-Dopa (which is converted to dopamine, a substance that is deficient in Parkinson's disease), but the method is enjoying a revival in the light of certain unsatisfactory aspects of L-Dopa. Although many patients on L-Dopa are able to move quicker and with more agility, the tremor often resists chemical amelioration, thus justifying in some instances the stereotactic procedure. In other cases, ultrasonic beams and radioactive substances have also been used to destroy brain tissue thought to be responsible for the tremors.

A major advance in the last five years has been the combining of stereotaxis with electrical stimulation to critical areas of the limbic system. Because the patient is awake during the treatment, he can describe the effects of the electrical stimulation. If stimulation of a certain area is found to reproduce symptoms for which treatment is sought (rage, depression, etc.), that area can be destroyed. This method has been used for years with good results in the treatment of epilepsy. Its value in treating behavioral disorders, however, has never been established.

Scientific publications regarding psychosurgical operations number many thousands by now. They are, for the most part, contradictory, confusing, and marred by the absence of scientific objectivity. Yet, despite the confusion and contradictions and, occasionally, downright deception, certain facts have emerged. For one thing, tampering with the frontal fibers is almost certain to produce indifference and apathy. This can be seen as well in diseases affecting the frontal lobes. One of my own patients with a ruptured blood vessel in the prefrontal area lost interest in his work and became careless and neglectful at home. His behavior and manner are now indistinguishable from many of the early lobotomy patients. In essence, any disease process affecting the prefrontal areas can be expected to produce a similar result.

So, too, with diseases affecting the limbic system. Limbic encephalitis, a viral disease involving parts of the limbic system, is marked by hallucinations, delusions, and violent agitation. Many of these patients are treated as if their strange behavior were due to nonorganic "functional" disorders. Later, when unmistakable signs of brain disease appear, the true nature of the condition is appreciated, often too late for anything to be done. Limbic encephalitis is in fact a paradigm of the ever narrowing gap between psychiatric disease on the one hand and organic disease of the nervous system on the other. With recognition of the vital part that brain function *must* play in behavior has come a resurgence of interest in altering behavior by altering the brain. Psychosurgery's ability to do this has been at best extremely spotty. Certain patients have reacted poorly to psychosurgery regardless of the type of operation. Schizophrenics have done worst of all and have been eliminated from the patient pool of even the most enthusiastic psychosurgeons. So-called psychopaths or sociopaths have not done much better.

Confusing as things are in the use of psychosurgery for distinct psychiatric illnesses, the waters are even more muddied when psychosurgery is applied for the control of violent or aggressive behavior. Animal studies over the last twenty years have resulted in the discovery that "aggression" or "violence" can be understood only in reference to the experimental situation in which it is displayed. Predatory aggression, for instance, refers to the tendency of rats to kill mice placed in the cage with them. Shock-induced aggression, on the other hand, refers to the likelihood of two animals attacking one another under the influence of periodic electric shocks. Both are "aggressive" and "violent" behaviors, but here the similarities end. Animals demonstrating predatory aggression often cannot be made to attack or become "violent" by means of electric shock, and the reverse is also true. In addition, sophisticated biochemical analysis demonstrates that different anatomical pathways and biochemical substances are involved in the different experimentally induced "violent" behaviors. Even the responses to medications vary, with tranquilizers working for some forms of "violence" while making others worse. The situation is similar in humans. Every physician is familiar with the so-called paradoxical response in which tranquilizers, instead of exerting a calming effect on a patient, result in even more violence and agitation. Aggression is aggression is aggression—another scientific platitude unmasked. Not surprisingly then, no one has come up with a foolproof psychosurgical operation specifically to reduce violence, since *violence* and *aggression* are meaningless terms outside of a defining social situation. In addition, many of the operations result in greater or lesser effects on intelligence, ambition, or just plain zest for living.

The earliest surgical attempts to control violence were on aggressive epileptics. Over the years, most of the epileptics operated on suffered from epilepsy involving the temporal lobe, which lies immediately alongside the amygdala and hippocampus with direct and two-way connections with the limbic system. Deeply placed electrodes sometimes detect in aggressive patients abnormal electrical discharges that originate in the temporal lobe and extend into the nearby limbic system. The patient's description of the events preceding a seizure often gives clues to the path of discharge. "Butterflies" in the stomach or "dizziness" may be the forewarning of a generalized grand mal attack, suggesting that the abnormal discharge has spread to the cerebral cortex. On other occasions the dizziness may give way to an agonizing sense of fear— "visceral fear"—literally paralyzing the patient with a nameless dread of the unknown. It is postulated that the response to such fears, as well as the resulting confusion after a seizure, trigger the violent or aggressive behavior; still, temporal-lobe epileptics are not *necessarily* violent. The accumulated medical experience with uncontrollable temporal-lobe epileptics documents a tendency for many of them to progress over the years into a psychotic state indistinguishable from schizophrenia. The "visceral fears" are elaborated into a delusional system in which powerful and malignant agents are believed to control the patient for sinister purposes. Competent psychiatrists examining patients like these often fail to distinguish on clinical grounds alone the temporal-lobe epileptics from schizophrenics. In this group, where epilepsy and psychosis coexist, severe behavioral disorders that often culminate in violence coexist with epileptic seizures. The usefulness of psychosurgery with such patients is the subject of an ongoing and often contentious debate.

The man who has contributed most to the advances in psychosurgery for victims of this schizophrenic type of temporal-lobe epilepsy is Murray A. Falconer, a grandfatherly, white-haired New Zealander who operates at the Maudesley Hospital in London. Dr. Falconer recently published an account in the *New England Journal of Medicine* of his twenty years' experience on surgery for temporal-lobe epileptics. His contribution to the ongoing debate about violence and epilepsy is to demonstrate that abnormalities occur rather consistently in the hippocampus of aggressive epileptics. (Among his patient population are a small but significant number in whom seizures and violent behavior coexist.) The abnormality is medial temporal sclerosis—a fancy way of saying a loss of brain cells in a special part of the hippocampus known as Ammon's Horn (named after the man who first described it). After surgery, 80 per cent of the patients operated on were improved in terms of psychosis and violence.

As a result of Dr. Falconer's work, some doctors have made extrapolations to say that certain types of abnormal behavior in temporal-lobe epilepsy might improve with surgery. From this it is only a step to postulating that behavioral problems *alone* justify surgery, even when the epileptic's seizures are controlled by medication. Others disagree violently—hence the debate whether surgery has any place in the control of violent behavior. At the root of this disagreement is our primitive and incomplete knowledge of the brain pathways involved in violent behavior. "At this time there is no unanimity of opinion concerning the morphophysiological substrates which underlie abnormal aggressive behavior in animals or man," concludes a recent National Institute of Mental Health report on *The Research Aspects of a Neurological Basis of Aggressive (Violent) Behavior.*

Combined with uncertainties about the brain pathways are the widely varying skills of psychosurgeons, who range from icepick wielders to master technicians with international reputations. As a result of these discrepancies, the whole issue of psychosurgery has recently come under legal challenges of violation of medical ethics and of the individual patient's civil rights.

The Law
and
Julio Martinez

Despite the implications of psychosurgery as an irreversible operation on the brain—the physical basis for the mind, the person, and the "soul"—only two court cases involving psychosurgery are on record. In one of them, a court in Pittsburgh, Pennsylvania, authorized surgery in 1947 as a "rehabilitative measure" on a prison inmate, Millard Wright, convicted for ten house break-ins and robberies. After surgery a different presiding judge decided against Wright's release, opting instead for reduction in his prison sentence. Despondent, Wright later took his life. From 1947 until July 1973 the legal issues remained unclarified because psychosurgery did not come to another court test. Could a prisoner have psychosurgery, as in Wright's case, as a precondition for his release? Most legal authorities thought he could not. A tougher question remained, however: Suppose the requested psychosurgery was not tied to release, parole, or increase in privileges? What are the prisoner's rights to avail himself of a treatment that might help him?

That question, too, has now been settled in the courts, at least in Michigan. In 1955 Louis Smith was sentenced to Ionia State Hospital after being found guilty of a brutal sex slaying of a student nurse. From the beginning of his sentence, Smith's behavior in the hospital was not violent or aggressive in any way. Finally, in May 1972, when Smith was within a year of release after eighteen years of confinement, the superintendent asked him to consider volunteering for a newly funded research program investigating the results of surgical treatment on "severe, uncontrollable, aggressive outbursts." An early release from the prison hospital or a gain in hospital privileges was not offered to him in return; that is, no coercion or persuasive pressure was put on him. Smith agreed in writing and was to be the first of twelve inmates to undergo surgery. Two months later, a suit filed by the Medical Committee for Human Rights in collaboration with the National Law Center in Washington, D.C., questioned the validity of Smith's consent: "It is clear from the record in this case that Smith's competence for making the decision concerning psychosurgery was impaired by the environment in which he has lived for so long and by the complexity of the issues; that Smith did not have sufficient information to consent knowingly; and that his consent was not voluntary because the hospital setting was apparently coercive and the desire for release inevitably shaped his decision." One thing supporting the Committee's contention was Smith's later withdrawal of consent when his further detention was declared unconstitutional.

In a landmark state decision, a three-judge panel decided psychosurgery could not be performed on the involuntarily confined. The concepts of prisons and mental hospitals as "inherently coercive" was supported. "We therefore conclude that involuntarily detained mental patients cannot give informed and adequate consent to experimental psychosurgical procedures on the brain." The door was not shut completely, however, on future applications to the involuntarily confined. The decision rested on "the state of medical knowledge as of the time of the writing of the opinion." The court left open the possibility that with further refinements in psychosurgical technique and a shift from experimental to commonly accepted neurosurgical procedure "involuntarily detained mental patients could consent to such an operation." For the present, however, psychosurgery on the involuntarily confined seems clearly prohibitive.

The Ionia State Hospital case, although a lower court decision, was an important one if for no other reason than its status as the first judicial pronouncement relating to psychosurgery and the involuntarily confined. But an equally important and more far-reaching decision now must be made about informed consent outside of institutional settings. As a response to the Ionia State Hospital case and to generally unfavorable publicity about psychosurgery, several institutions have recently called for a moratorium; since March 1973 the federal government has canceled all funding of psychosurgery. A bill introduced in the Ninety-third Congress, first session, by Ohio Congressman Louis Stokes seeks "to prohibit psychosurgery in federally connected health care facilities." All these developments suggest a national move toward the total outlawing of psychosurgery. Some people, however, worry that such a measure may set a dangerous precedent by forcing the law into the position of practicing medicine.

To George J. Annas, director for the Center of Law and Health Sciences at the Boston University School of Law, this is undesirable and probably unnecessary. According to Dr. Annas, the necessary protections against irresponsible psychosurgery already exist. What is needed rather than blanket prohibition is an intelligent use of currently available legal restraints. Dr. Annas speaks of two legal avenues available to regulate psychosurgery: the private and the public. He has indicated how appropriate regulation could have been carried out even with the earliest psychosurgical procedures: "In any surgery the surgeon is under the obligation to provide the average standard of care, that is, he must perform as well as other surgeons doing the same operation. He must also have the same qualifications. This certainly would have eliminated the 3500 icepick lobotomies performed by Walter Freeman, who wasn't even a surgeon. If Freeman were doing that procedure now he would be in jail." The second standard suggested by Dr. Annas is that the operation be done without negligence. A case recently settled out of court involved a psychosurgeon who accidently cut the optic nerve, leading to total blindness in one eye. "This was obviously negligence. It is not a common nor acceptable complication for this kind of surgery."

But the most pointed objection to psychosurgery rests on the matter of the validity of informed consent: the extent to which the patient has been informed regarding all possible consequences of the psychosurgery. According to Dr. Annas, "The patient has an absolute right to self-decision. If he's going to have an operation on his back, for instance, and the surgeon doesn't tell him that there's a one per cent risk of paralysis, that constitutes an uninformed consent. In the same way he's got to be told everything that might happen to him as a consequence of having psychosurgery."

Some psychosurgeons think Annas's requirements may be impossible to attain in the light of changes brought about by the depth electrode techniques that are widely used prior to psychosurgery. For example, a patient of Dr. Vernon Mark, "Thomas the engineer," consented to psychosurgery while under the influence of electrical stimulation. Later, when the affects of the stimulus wore off, he refused consent; surgery was carried out anyway. Now the guardian of Thomas R. is suing Dr. Mark. Thomas R., meanwhile, remains in a state hospital, reported "intellectually deteriorated" and unable to manage his everyday affairs. Could Thomas R. give an "informed consent" to have a brain operation when he was under the influence of electrical stimulation?

An increasing number of civil libertarians think that the basic legal problem stems from a lack of regulation of surgeons in general. While the Food and Drug Administration regulates all prescription medications used in the United States, no such regulating agency exists for surgeons other than their own specialty boards. Even now, more than a third of the general surgeons in the United States are "surgeons" by self-designation rather than training or specialty certification. "This is the kind of setting we have here in the United States," Dr. Annas has said. "It's not surprising that the psychosurgeon's studies are anecdotal and unscientific. They usually report on the results of their own surgery, which of course is patently ridiculous. Both the patient and the surgeon have an interest in reporting a cure." This present legal embroil can probably be expected to become even more complex in the light of a new neurosurgical technique developed just recently. No less than the very definition of psychosurgery may have to be changed.

Julio Martinez had his first seizure when he was six months old. After a workup at a major medical center in New York found no cause for the incident, Julio was placed on an anticonvulsant that only partially helped him; he continued to have weekly, sometimes even daily seizures. By the time he was ten his major seizures alternated with brief staring episodes, which often were followed by sudden outbursts of unprovoked destructive behavior. His major attacks, grand mal, lasted from two to eight minutes and occurred once a day or every other day. He also reported sensations of anger, hostility, and depression. In his teens Julio made several attempts at suicide, once by shooting himself in the chest with a rifle, once by an overdose of barbiturates, once by savagely slashing his wrists until restrained by his parents. He dropped out of school, spent his time wandering aimlessly around the neighborhood, and got into innumerable fights. During one episode of rage when he was eighteen, he smashed all the furniture in his house and tried to kill his mother. At this point his parents were desperate for anything that could help Julio.

So far, Julio Martinez's plight is no different from that of many others who over the years have eventually been persuaded to undergo one or another form of psychosurgery. If this were 1943, Walter Freeman might well plunge an icepick into Julio's frontal lobes. Even two years ago a neurosurgical operation would have placed the tiny stereotactic lesions in his amygdala. In both instances irreversible destruction of brain tissue would have resulted. But Julio's treatment in February 1973 was new and innovative; he was among the first of thirty-four patients operated on by Dr. Irving Cooper of St. Barnabas Hospital in New York City for the implantation of a cerebellar electrical stimulator.

Our understanding of the contribution of the cerebellum to the total functioning of the brain has recently undergone a profound change. A small, three-lobed structure behind the occipital lobes, the most posterior part of the cerebral cortex, the cerebellum is important to movement and coordination. When we reach for an apple, bring it to our mouth, bite, chew, and swallow a piece of it, the cerebellum is the brain structure that coordinates the thousands of separate muscle movements necessary. Without the cerebellum we would not be able to pick up the apple at all, or if we could, would not be able to stop our returning hand from smashing in our front teeth. For the cerebellum acts as a modulator, dampening out the tendency for each motor act, once started, to go on and on indefinitely. Once the hand starts toward the apple, something must be able to coordinate, perfect, and stop the motion when the apple has been grasped. That is one function of the cerebellum. Patients with cerebellar disease are unable to do such things as drink a cup of coffee because the cerebellum is no longer able to function as a coordinator. As a result, scalding burns may be inflicted as the hot liquid falls over hands and face. This is the classic understanding of the cerebellum, and so far, it seems to have little to offer either Julio's seizures or his violent outbursts.

To Dr. Cooper the cerebellum hinted at capabilities even more complex than the coordination of movements. Cooper dug into nineteenth-century neurophysiological reports to find experimental evidence that stimulation of the anterior lobe of the cerebellum could release "decerebrate rigidity," a diseased brain state resulting in the experimental animals' inability to move voluntarily. Such animals are literally "stiff as a board," and will remain so indefinitely. These early researchers had found that cerebellar stimulation reversed this rigid state. This suggested to Dr. Cooper and others that the cerebellum also functioned as a modulator of neurologic activity in the cerebral cortex, activity that is abnormally heightened in epilepsy.

Support for this concept of the cerebellum's "gating effect" on the brain came from Dr. Robert S. Dow at the Laboratory of Neurophysiology, Good Samaritan Medical Center,

Portland, Oregon. Dr. Dow showed that epileptic seizures in cats could be aborted by cerebellar stimulation. Further, epileptic waves that failed to produce a seizure could be made to disappear entirely at selected frequencies of cerebellar stimulation. According to Dr. Dow, "The concept of chronic cerebellar stimulation is based on a thesis that the Purkinje cell [the specialized cerebellar brain cell bringing about inhibition] can be prosthetically induced to modify neurologic activity which is abnormally heightened as in a seizure."

Cautiously and with scrupulous attention to the issue of informed consent, Dr. Cooper set out in early 1973 to try out a cerebellar stimulator in cases of severe and otherwise untreatable epilepsy. One of the first of these was Julio Martinez.

"Once we started stimulation, he had no grand mal or psychomotor seizures, though there were several seizures in the twenty-four hours after implantation before stimulation started," Dr. Cooper reported. For two and a half months after surgery Julio did well, experiencing neither a seizure nor a rage outburst. Then one night, after a drinking spree, Julio broke a wire in the stimulator and had thirteen major seizures; the next day the wire was repaired by Dr. Cooper and Julio has been seizure-free ever since. Perhaps more importantly, the rage episodes have stopped altogether, enabling Julio to hold his first job, as a machinist's apprentice.

As Dr. Cooper is quick to point out, Julio Martinez's operation was not psychosurgery. There was "no surgical removal or destruction of brain tissue to disconnect one part of the brain from another with the intent of altering behavior," as psychosurgery is defined by Dr. Bertram Brown, director of the National Institute of Mental Health. And Julio is no longer destroying furniture and wandering the streets, ready at any time to explode into a senseless and dangerous rage. In its overall results, therefore, the cerebellar-stimulation technique may turn out to be more effective than any psychosurgical operation yet devised.

According to Dr. Michael Riklon, director of the Department of Psychology at St. Barnabas, "A cerebellar role has now been shown in perception and behavior. Cerebellar stimulation influences levels of excitability in sensory areas of the cerebral cortex. Stimulation of the audio-visual area, for instance, provokes responses in both auditory and visual cortical areas. These indications of possible cerebellar influences on higher integrated behavioral functions lead us to question the effects of stimulation on these functions."

At least for now, the exact mechanism that lies behind Julio's improvement remains unknown. Dr. Cooper postulates that chemical effects may be induced by the stimulation, leading to a type of brain reconditioning. If this is what happens, the cerebellar-stimulation technique may be actually curing rather than just controlling Julio's symptoms. Someday, Dr. Cooper may even test this hypothesis by removing the stimulator, with the hope that the seizures or violent behavior will not recur.

Cerebellar-stimulation techniques have not been applied to patients who do not have demonstrably abnormal brain tissue similar to Julio's; nor are there any plans at this point to do so. But obviously the technique gets around some of the most forceful legal objections to psychosurgery: brain tissue is not destroyed; the operation is not irreversible; the stimulation can be initiated by the patient himself and remains under his control, thus obviating the robotlike effects of earlier psychosurgery. In addition, "informed consent" is not so urgent because the operation is safer and more predictable in its effect. And if things don't work out, the stimulator can be removed by a minor operation and everybody returns to square one.

What would be the legal status of such an operation if somebody eventually gets around to using it for a purely behavioral problem? "I think this operation just blows the whole psychosurgery question wide open," commented one lawyer who specializes in the legal issues of behavior-control techniques. "The use of this operation will circumvent most of the objections to traditionally irreversible psychosurgical procedures. It will even soften the consent issue because informed consent is obviously easier to get with a less dangerous and totally reversible operation." If nothing else, the cerebellar-stimulation technique makes clear that prohibitive laws are not the answer. In the future, newer and subtler technologies may bring us closer to a situation anticipated by philosopher Robert Neville: "If a helpful and safe psychosurgical procedure is discovered, we can't put ourselves in the position of depriving a patient of his right to treatment particularly if the prohibition is based on laws drawn up now, when our ignorance factor regarding the human brain is so colossal."

A Way Out

Within the last few years a possible solution to the bioethical issues raised by psychosurgery has been put into operation at Harvard University, based on the concept of community involvement in medical decision making. The plan is the brainchild of Dr. David F. Allen, Kennedy Fellow in Medical Ethics at Harvard University. While a resident in psychiatry at the Harvard Medical School, Dr. Allen was fascinated by the furious and often bitter controversy surrounding Dr. Vernon Mark's psychosurgery at the Boston City Hospital (which I shall discuss further; see below, p. 28). In early 1973 Dr. Allen approached the administrator of the hospital with his plan.

By his own admission, Dr. Allen, a black psychiatrist who hails from Nassau in the Bahamas, had been "lost in the anatomic details involved in psychosurgery." If he, as a physician, found it difficult to sort out all the details, Dr. Allen reasoned, it must be almost impossible for those without training in medicine or surgery to evaluate any psychosurgical operation; and the medical input alone obviously wasn't enough.

Dr. Allen's plan was deceptively simple. He suggested a multidisciplinary review committee be established at Harvard and the Boston City Hospital to review all psychosurgical operations. The committee should be composed of a theologian, a lawyer, a sociologist, a psychologist, a neurologist, and a neurosurgeon, as well as other members of the community. After some initial friction, this idea eventually received the support of the administrator and the cooperation of Dr. Mark. All patients considered for psychosurgery were first to appear before the committee, whose members would question them freely to determine such matters as the adequacy of their consent and the appropriateness of their selection. In the end, the committee would decide whether or not psychosurgery should be performed. Both the administrator and Dr. Mark agreed that the committee should have veto powers: if it decided psychosurgery should not be done, the surgeon agreed not to carry it out.

"In the beginning I don't think many of us on the committee realized the tremendous responsibility we were assuming," said Dr. Allen. "But at some time during our interviews, it hit all of us: 'I am going to have to make a decision whether or not this guy is going to have brain surgery.' Even as a physician, I don't like making these kinds of decisions. You can imagine how the others felt." Dr. Allen noticed that many of the committee's members tried to find ways of avoiding a final decision. The attorney, for instance, recommended an advocacy situation in which somebody could summarize the case in favor of psychosurgery and somebody else could develop a case against it. The sociologist suggested that the decision be put off until the committee had a chance to visit the patient's home and work situation and until more data were available. A clergyman thought the decision should be postponed until a report was sent from the hospital chaplain. "Everybody fell back into his own particular professional role. We all knew that we could never know everything that might be important in arriving at a decision." Dr. Allen compared the committee's job to a jury assignment. "Sure, it would be great for a jury to be able to go to the scene of an accident and interview everybody concerned and see the accident reconstructed, etc., but this isn't practical or even possible. In real life you have to make some important decisions on admittedly incomplete data."

As I write, Allen's committee has been meeting for less than six months; during that time, it has not been called upon to make as many decisions as some members would like—in fact, since Dr. Mark's psychosurgical operations are quite infrequent, only four times. The first patient to appear, a man with a history of violent outbursts, denied both the fact of his violence and the suggestion that anything at all was wrong. "For a few minutes we thought the wrong man had been brought into the committee room. He was quite polite and affirmed his denial that a problem existed." The committee decided psychosurgery was not indicated in this instance since informed consent couldn't possibly be achieved. "Do you know what happened next?" Dr. Allen recalls. "Two weeks later he was arrested after a shooting spree during which, luckily, no one was hurt. Were we wrong in not recommending psychosurgery in his case? I don't know, but that man haunts me."

The second patient was evaluated as an exercise for the committee after surgery had already been performed. "We wanted to see what the results were. In this case—which was similar to the first, with frequent episodes of disorderly conduct and repeated brushes with the law—the surgery was both success and failure. By that I mean he hasn't been in any more legal entanglements but he is not happy with himself and to that extent the operation was a failure."

Dr. Allen sees his role as mediator between medicine and society. "My aim is to bring these technical issues into the mainstream of society, and work with it in a democratic framework." What is most to be feared, he thinks, is the maintenance of "privilege groups." "Technology without an educated public is ethically untenable because it results in privilege groups that feel that they alone have the knowledge and others have no knowledge." Dr. Allen is quick to point out that he is not advocating doing away with expert opinion. He would just like to broaden things enough to draw from presently unutilized areas of expertise. "Society can no longer stand back and wait for something to be done. Each member of society has a contribution here. Our committee is saying, in effect, 'Come with us and let's look at this thing together because we're all part of the same society.' It's a societal concept really—a societal responsibility."

Although it has been in operation only a short time, some people are suggesting that Dr. Allen's multidisciplinary review panel be used as a model across the nation. It provides education for the patient regarding the full implications of his proposed surgery; support for the family; even support for the surgeon (in case of later charges of malpractice). Others, however, are urging a more cautious optimism. "I think total satisfaction at this point with the review panel will be premature," the psychosurgeon Dr. Mark says. "The committee is entering into the practice of medicine, and we can't just slide over the implications of this." Dr. Mark wants to clarify whether the committee is responsible for the decisions it makes. Some patients referred to it for psychosurgery have had long histories of violent behavior. "What kind of safeguards is the committee going to give to the community?" asks Dr. Mark. In addition, there is the question of licensing and determining who should sit on the committee. "As a surgeon my credentials are always up for examination and review. I don't want to see anything less than a qualified review for the members of this committee. Who's going to examine them and by what criteria?" Dr. Mark is also uneasy about the intrusion of political issues into the committee's decisions. "If people are sick they should not be denied treatment just because of some political philosophy which says all psychosurgery is totalitarian or fascist."

Still, although major practical issues remain unresolved, the cooperation of surgeons with Dr. Allen's committee has brought about at least a mutual respect. As one committee member puts it, "If we can't reach a decision with all the varied expertise on this committee, then maybe we should be less critical of Dr. Mark, who has somehow had to decide everything on his own. Believe me, the decisions are anguishing." The multidisciplinary review committee is obviously not perfect. Besides, it still awaits a real test of fire. If events in the next year indicate a broadening acceptance and funding for psychosurgery, the committee may be called upon to make tougher and tougher decisions. But to my mind it is still probably the best approach to developing ethical controls in psychosurgery. "Some type of review committee is an absolute must" Dr. Annas has said. "The committee must be represented in such decisions which are not strictly medical." Dr. Annas compares the present situation to events prior to the development of the atomic bomb. "Along with the physicists at Oak Ridge there should have been something like this committee which has more of an overview than just the technical-scientific."

Whether or not the review committee idea survives, some measure of control over psychosurgery is obviously needed. Reliance on the strictly medical model is proving dreadfully inefficient, combining as it does barbarically crude conceptions of the brain and of behavior with childishly naive notions of the nature of informed consent. Nor are the problems likely to disappear in the near future. Technologically induced behavior modification is proving to be this century's most compelling medical social issue. Current fads for ESP and biofeedback reflect our enthusiasm for controlling mental processes with techniques similar to those for controlling our physical environment. Psychosurgery, the most extreme and dramatic form of such modification, involves particularly anguishing decisions that must be made *now*. Further, as I have tried to make clear, far more complex issues are involved than simply "medical" or "scientific" decisions. No less is at stake than the use of biotechnology for the purpose of social control. It seems to me certain measures are justified and urgently needed.

First, it is time for a temporary moratorium on all forms of psychosurgery undertaken primarily to modify behavior. The social and political consequences of allowing behavioral scientists and surgeons to act as social engineers has not been sufficiently thought through. As I shall show in the following sections on behavior modification, the question is not so much "how to control behavior" as it is "who is to be the controller and who is to be the controlled."

Second, we need a clearinghouse of information on the effects of brain lesions on behavior. As things stand, the facts are scattered in hundreds of articles in medical journals and other learned papers. A clearinghouse would enable us to evaluate the data already accumulated over twenty years from various psychosurgical procedures. Dr. Robert Neville has recently suggested a national registry of all psychosurgical procedures performed in the past. This could be combined with the clearinghouse data.

Third, from here it should be possible to determine national standards of practice concerning a number of vital issues: when and if psychosurgery is indicated; what procedures offer reasonable hope of effective results; most importantly, what patients are eligible for psychosurgery and under what circumstances.

Fourth, we must have ways to protect the individual patient from having psychosurgical procedures imposed upon him against his will or in a setting in which his informed consent or capacity to choose is impaired. This means proxy consent will not be allowed, nor will psychosurgery be performed on incompetent medical patients or the involuntarily detained, whether in hospitals or in prisons.

Finally, since the results of psychosurgery have not been established, all psychosurgical procedures should be considered experimental and subject to strictly imposed controls. Operations should be carried out only in a clinical institution able to provide total therapeutic care and follow-up. Nonmedical disciplines must have a significant influence in the control of psychosurgery. The medical profession's contribution can be used to best advantage in the evaluation of scientific protocols, since physicians can best interpret their scientific validity. Beyond that, particularly with regard to the social and legal issues surrounding psychosurgery, physicians' and scientists' contributions are valuable, but no more so than that of any reflective citizen.

The alternative, of course, is simply to do away with psychosurgery once and for all. But even this drastic total prohibition isn't as simple as it seems. What is to be done for the tortured compulsives whose senseless rituals defy treatment by any other form? What of the terminal cancer patient whose personality threatens to shatter under the daily strain of unendurable pain? These people can be helped by limited forms of psychosurgery. Even granting for the moment that other psychiatric treatments are preferable for compulsions and intractable pain, what is to be done for patients who freely request a psychosurgical procedure? What are their rights? At this point, these questions cannot be answered for want of facts. With facts can come *meaningful* regulation and control. "Many medical abuses are less the consequences of oppressive control than of lack of control," Dr. Annas has remarked. "The horrifying truth is that now no one is in charge."

The Biotechnology of Repression: The Beginning

Obviously psychosurgery is definitive and irreversible. Because of its finality, the question of how it should be used is understandably stirring up dramatic debate. But no less critical are other methods of behavior control already in use in various parts of the United States. The issue of behavior control, whether by psychosurgery or other means, cannot be understood intelligently without reference to issues far removed from scientific considerations. In fact, much more can be gained from considering behavior control within the broader context of currently unresolved social conflicts.

It is not coincidental that behavior-control technology received its greatest support from the same government administration that provided us with Watergate. Partly in reaction to campus unrest and racial confrontation in the late 1960s, the government's interest in the control of "violence" reached almost monomaniacal proportions that led to dubious and threatening collaborations between government agencies and behavior-control scientists. As we head into the future, greater and greater numbers of us are likely to become targets for behavior control. Already the hardware is here for manipulating our behavior. Even more frightening than hardware is the absence of any ethical or social constraints on the work of behavior scientists. Moreover, in the last several years many scientists have allowed their work to be funded and directed by government agencies that are less interested in science than they are in the social control and manipulation of disturbingly large numbers of us.

The story of this strange alliance between the government and behavioral scientists began in 1967 with a letter to the editor of the *Journal of the American Medical Association*. Its authors—Vernon Mark, from the Department of Neurosurgery at the Boston City Hospital; Frank Ervin, a Harvard psychiatrist; and William Sweet, chief of neurosurgery at Massachusetts General Hospital—suggested a new and different way of viewing the Watts riots. In "The Role of Brain Disease in Riots and Urban Violence" they wrote: "It is important to realize that only a small number of the millions of slum dwellers have taken part in the riots and that only a subfraction of these rioters have indulged in arson, sniping and assault. And if slum conditions alone determined the initiated riots, why are the vast majority of slum dwellers able to resist the temptations of unrestrained violence? Is there something peculiar about the violent slum dweller that differentiates him from his peaceful neighbor?" The group called attention to "the more subtle role of other possible factors, including brain dysfunction in the rioters who engaged in arson, sniping and physical assault." The letter ended with the statement of a set of goals that were to prove of compelling interest to a government preoccupied with violence and the threat of violence: "We need intensive research and clinical studies of the *individual* committing the violence. The goals of such studies would be to pinpoint, diagnose, and treat those people with low violence thresholds before these contribute to further tragedies."

Over the next three years Drs. Mark, Sweet, and Ervin continued their search for clinical methods of detecting and treating violent people. Together they formed the Neuro Research Foundation which, in 1970, was contacted by the newly established Law Enforcement Assistance Administration (LEAA) of the Department of Justice. Through the LEAA a $109,000 grant was funneled into the Foundation for the purpose of developing studies to identify "violence-prone individuals." Thus was begun an elaborate and ominous collaboration between the government and behavior scientists that was unprecedented both in scope and implication. Looking back now, several years later, it seems the most obvious question was not asked: why was an agency in the Department of Justice becoming involved in neurosurgical studies on violence? The answer to that can be found, I believe, by checking some of the background facts on why the LEAA was created.

In 1968 the passage of the Omnibus Crime Control and Safe Streets Act was the first major effort to provide "large-scale financial assistance for the prevention and reduction of crime at the state and city level." As part of that Act, the LEAA was created for the purpose of providing funds to states for "local crime prevention and reduction programs." Included in the purposes of LEAA were research in law enforcement and criminal justice, as well as educational assistance for law-enforcement personnel. Nowhere in the Omnibus Crime Control and Safe Streets Act or the Law Enforcement Assistance Act (which created LEAA) was any mention made of an intended purpose to support such activities as the study of violence prevention or the development of techniques of behavior modification. One may also note that at the time the government created LEAA it cut back drastically on funds available to medical research through traditional channels such as the NIH, thus creating a mad scramble for other sources of research support. One of the most attractive sources seemed to be LEAA.

To appreciate how totally inappropriate the LEAA funding was, it is necessary to compare it with the usual funding procedures. Over the years scientists have developed an elaborate system for obtaining government support for research known as peer review. This basically consists of a group of scientists reviewing all research proposals that come to the government and judging them on their scientific merit. Those that are judged scientifically meritorious are funded, in the form of federal grants. Now it goes without saying that this traditional practice depends on a high degree of sophistication in the people who evaluate research proposals. They need to be and are scientists with whatever background or training is required to recognize a sound scientific proposal when they see one. In the case of LEAA, no such peer review was possible because those approving the Neuro Research Foundation proposals were not scientists and knew absolutely nothing about either neurosurgery or the neurological basis of aggression. Not surprisingly, with this as a standard operating procedure, LEAA came under a lot of criticism.

In response to congressional pressures, an independent peer review of the work of the Neuro Research Foundation led to discontinuance of LEAA funding. The reviewers concluded: "Despite its bulk, this study contributes relatively little to our knowledge of biological factors in violence. The authors have not found test procedures that identify the violent criminals and the methods used . . . do not hold out much hope that this can be done by them."

In 1970 Drs. Mark and Ervin published a book entitled *Violence and the Brain* with a foreword by Dr. Sweet stating the book's principal thesis: "Human behavior, including assaultive action, is an expression of the functioning brain." By studying violent persons with recognizable brain disease, the group hypothesized knowledge "that can be applied to combat the violence triggered mechanisms in the brain of the non-diseased." In this book, as in the earlier research proposal made to the LEAA, the tantalizing prospect of *prediction* of violent behavior was held out, that "tests may be developed to detect at an early stage the person with poor control of dangerous impulses is an especially appealing likelihood."

By the end of 1971 not only had the Neuro Research Foundation lost its LEAA funding, but in response to further congressional pressures, Dr. Sweet was asked to appear before a Subcommittee on Appropriations to answer questions about his request for a million dollars to continue his research. Under stiff questioning, Dr. Sweet called the work done so far a "success" but did not submit a report or a summary of research activities carried out by the Foundation. After lengthy debate, Dr. Sweet's million-dollar proposal was denied. With the loss of both LEAA and NIH funding, any further research into the supposed biological foundations of violence seemed doomed. Other events were occurring, however, that would serve to inject new life into the search for the biological basis of violence.

The Search for an End to Violence

In 1969 Dr. Louis Jolyon West came to UCLA from the University of Oklahoma "to look into the act of pathological violence, that which is usually committed against members of one's own family or neighbors." As the new chairman of the Department of Psychiatry at UCLA and director of its Neuropsychiatric Institute, Dr. West, or "Jolly," as he is known to his friends, brought with him an international reputation for his earlier studies on violence among American Indians. West had also specialized in the psychiatric investigation of violent criminals (the most famous of his patients was Jack Ruby).

In September 1972 Dr. West drew up a proposal written in collaboration with Dr. J. M. Stubblebine, director of the state's Department of Health. In it he called for the establishment at UCLA of a new permanent Center for the Prevention of Violence. Over the next five years West was to ask for a million dollars a year; the initial figure requested in his grant was simply a million dollars for the first year. His plans called for the completion by July 1, 1973, of the first phase of the Center at UCLA in "close cooperation with various agencies of the State of California—including correction and law enforcement." The Center's ultimate objectives as defined in West's proposal were to develop "reliable predictors and/or determinates of some types of violent behavior so that it becomes possible to predict the probability of occurrence of types of violent behavior and *to identify certain individuals who are characterized by a very high probability of committing individual acts of violence."* (Italics mine.)

The parallels between West's project and the earlier Neuro Research work of Drs. Ervin, Mark, and Sweet are striking. But the similarities did not stop with a shared commitment to identifying potentially violent people. For one thing, money for Dr. West's Violence Center was to come ultimately from the state of California, via the California Council for Criminal Justice (CCCJ), the California branch of LEAA. For another, the loss of Dr. Sweet's million dollars coincided with Dr. West's proposal to obtain the same amount for similar research from the CCCJ. Finally, Dr. Frank Ervin resigned his position at Boston and, at the invitation of Dr. West, joined the faculty of UCLA's Department of Psychiatry to carry out a proposal entitled "Violence and the Brain: Bioelectrical and Behavioral Studies."

Although Dr. West's grant application to a division of the Department of Justice was unique in California legislation, precedent existed within the state for cooperative projects between law-enforcement or penal agencies and mental-health professionals. In fact, one of the prison facilities mentioned as a "satellite" hospital in Dr. West's proposal, Atascadero State Hospital for the Criminally Insane, had received national headlines three years earlier for its use of a form of treatment known as aversion therapy.*

---

* In late 1968 three mental-health professionals on the staff at Atascadero published their results on succinylcholine, a drug capable of producing total body paralysis and respiratory arrest without loss of consciousness. The overall effect of succinylcholine has been described as "a sensation of suffocation akin to drowning," or in the words of the investigators: "Succinylcholine produces a decidedly unpleasant and fearful sensation during which the sensorium is intact and the patient rendered susceptible to suggestion." Indeed, "suggestion" formed the basis of a succinylcholine aversion "treatment." With the patient completely paralyzed and his respiration supported, a therapist loomed overhead intoning suggestions for improved behavior and spelling out in no uncertain terms the penalties for further misbehavior. As the drug wore off, within three to five minutes, the treatment ceased and the prisoners returned to their cells, many of them "vastly improved." In December 1969 the hospital staff was ordered to stop the succinylcholine treatment altogether, pending the submission of a research protocol acceptable to the Department of Mental

Now to the actual working proposal for the Violence Center. Dr. West's proposal of September 1972 was only the first of six drafts drawn up over six months in response to mounting criticism. The first one focused on "violent individuals who because of biological, emotional or characterological disturbances are prone to life-threatening behavior." I have obtained copies of several of the proposed studies that were to be sponsored by the Violence Center. They include:

■ "The Sexually Violent Male." This study was to be based on the hypothesis that violent, especially sexually violent, behavior could be traced to fluctuations in the levels of the male sex hormones, the androgens. A test drug, cyproterone acetate, was reported by European laboratories as producing "a temporary, safe, and reversible partial inhibition of androgen metabolism." It was postulated that the drug's mechanism of action depended on its blocking effect on the sex hormones, particularly in the brain. The study called for the selection and segregation of those in prison for violent sexual assaults and the forced aministration of cyproterone acetate. The proposal warned that "the investigation of cyproterone acetate may take months or years to complete" and "perhaps will never be accepted for use in this country for this purpose." Among the major needs of the study was "further testing of the chemical for effects on normal volunteers," a virtual admission that the total biological effects of cyproterone acetate still awaited definition. Most interesting of all was the suggestion that the study not necessarily be confined to the imprisoned. "Appropriate non-institutionalized clinical subjects suffering from violent sexual behavior must be identified." No suggestions

---

Hygiene research adviser council. In at least five instances the staff had authorized the treatment despite refusal of the prisoners to give consent.

Nor was Atascadero unique among California prisons in its use of various forms of behavior modification. The medical facility at Vacaville, a prison psychiatric institution, also carried out succinylcholine aversion therapy. In addition, at least three amygdalotomies were performed on prisoners before 1971, when further operations were forbidden by the Department of Corrections and the University of California. Both Atascadero and Vacaville were included in Dr. West's proposal as "appropriate locations throughout the state" where the Violence Center's actual studies would be carried out.

were made, however, as to how this identification was to be carried out, or how noninstitutionalized men would be induced to participate in the study.

■ "Chromosomal Factors and Violent Behavior." This study proposal begins by commenting on the association between violent behavior and the chromosomal abnormality XYY. In this rare condition, the male sex chromosome is doubled, resulting in XYY rather than the usual XY. Some investigators have reported an increased incidence of violence among those with the XYY genotype. In an attempt to study this further, their research proposal suggested the development of techniques for identifying subjects with the XYY makeup. Ultimately the study's objective was to find out "whether or not hormonal or neurohumoral transmitters mediate the predisposition to violent episodes." The proposal leaves out such intriguing questions as how the chromosomal determination would be carried out, on whom, and what would be done with the information. Despite these ambiguities, however, it concludes on the bureaucratically hopeful note of "a cost benefit analysis for carrying out a large-scale study of the XYY problem."

■ "Violence and Minimal Brain Damage in Children." Children with the so-called minimal-brain-damage syndrome demonstrate hyperactivity, poor concentration, reduced mental skills, motor restlessness, and difficulties in interpersonal relationships usually thought to be secondary to their overactivity. Despite the label of minimal brain damage, not all neurologists or educators are convinced that the condition is neurological or necessarily abnormal. The proposed study, however, referred to "clinical studies of certain violent adults suggesting that minimal brain dysfunction and its effects while growing up may have played a role in the genesis of their abnormal behavior." To appreciate just what is involved in this statement, it should be realized that widespread recognition of minimal brain damage dates back only twenty years at the most. If we assume that the average child was diagnosed at age seven or eight and followed into adulthood, then it is obvious that we are talking about one generation followed for no more than thirty years. The investigators, however, have accepted as a given the association of minimal brain damage and subsequent violent behavior! They call for "follow-up studies of the subject children and their families to determine which characteristics of hyperactive children correlate most with such behaviors as fighting, murder, threatening, fire-setting, assaults, self-mutilation and the like." Nowhere is any mention made of the actual methods that will be used to select the minimally brain damaged or whose definition will be employed. There is only this assertion: "It should be particularly noted that the subjects in this research have been subjected to meticulously careful differential diagnosis rather than the crude methods of assessment too often employed. . . . This study should add significantly to knowledge and effectiveness in the diagnosis, evaluation and preventive treatment of children with MBD who also have a high potential for the development of violent behavior."

Both "The Sexually Violent Male" and "Chromosomal Factors and Violent Behavior" are examples of proposed studies of captive populations: the inmates of prisons and mental institutions. Studies such as "Violence and Minimal Brain Damage in Children," however, introduced a new twist based on the investigation of people whose freedoms are not limited by commitment or imprisonment. In addition, the numbers of potential subjects for the Violence Center increased fantastically by the addition of studies such as that on alcoholism proposed by Dr. West. In proposal Number 1, September 1, 1972, he wrote: "Evidence is also mounting that predisposition to alcoholism may be inherited. Because of the notorious connection between alcoholism and violent behavior this avenue should be explored thoroughly. *Predisposed individuals* [italics mine] identified early enough could be prevented from developing alcoholism." Dr. West never elaborated on how future alcoholics were to be "identified early enough" or how alcoholism could be prevented.

One particularly intriguing study suggested by Dr. West was the use of remote monitoring techniques. Dr. West wrote, "It is even possible to record bioelectrical changes in the brain of freely moving subjects through the use of remote monitoring techniques. These methods now require elaborate preparation. They're not yet feasible for large-scale screening that might permit detection of violence predisposing brain disorders prior to the occurrence of a violent episode. The major task of the Center should be to derive such a test, perhaps sharpened in its predictive powers by correlated measures, psychological test results, biochemical changes in urine and blood, etc." Also included were plans for electrophysiologic methods of remote control of behavior by computer.

Dr. West's proposal was not the first to suggest electronic surveillance as a means of social control. Six years earlier, a Harvard psychologist, Ralph Schwitzgebel, had written of "the community as a laboratory" and called for such things as having mental patients wear two-way transmitters by which they could be located and controlled. Schwitzgebel called this "preventive social science." He said, "We may soon be reaching the point where it will be possible to allow some emotionally ill people the freedom of the streets provided they are effectively 'defused' through chemical agents. The task, then, for the computer-linked sensors would be to telemeter, not their emotional states, but simply the sufficiency of concentration of the chemical agent to insure an acceptable emotional state." In 1971 the NIMH published a monograph by Schwitzgebel (now unobtainable) entitled *Development and Legal Regulation of Coercive Behavior Mod Techniques with Offenders*. Although not specifically mentioned by Dr. West in the proposal, the Schwitzgebel monograph is the classic on "behavioral instrumentation."

Additional studies in Dr. West's first proposal, written in 1972, included "Biological Predicters in Early Childhood of Subsequent Impaired Impulse Control"; "Violence and the Brain: Bioelectrical and Behavioral Studies"; "Marijuana Use in Violent Behavior"; "Violence in the Hyperkinetic Child"; "Fire-Setting by Children"—in all, twenty proposals.

One approved and funded proposal involved subjects hospitalized as mentally disordered sex offenders (MDSO) entitled "Errorless Extinction of Deviant Sexual Interests." The study involved subjects, all men, sitting in a dimly lit room observing slides depicting "deviant sexual activity." As a measure of each man's sexual response to the slides, his penile engorgement was monitored by a mechanical strain gauge forming one part of an electronic circuit. After choosing the most sexually provocative slides, as measured by "penile engorgement," each subject was "instructed in a method to assist in the control of the sexual response." Suggested methods included "the substitution of incompatible intellectual responses, such as counting backwards, repeating song lyrics, etc., or covert sensitization where a maladaptive approach response is prevented from occurring by preceding it with imagined knocks of stimulus, such as nausea, vomiting, etc." In a letter to Bernard Weiner of the San Francisco *Chronicle,* Dr. Richard Laws, the investigator in charge of "Errorless Extinction of Deviant Sexual Interests," described in detail how the experiment would work. "Subjects will be shown pictures of persons they found sexually attractive, e.g., female child molesters would see pictures of little girls. On their penises they would have worn a lightweight, spring steel ring on the top of which is a wheatstone bridge circuit through which is passed a very weak electrical current. Any change in the size of the penis would unbalance this bridge and inverse the resistance of the circuit." The end result of all of this would be an electric shock to the genitals.

By late 1972, all was in readiness for a quick approval of funding for the Violence Center. In many cases, equipment had already been purchased for studies such as "Errorless Extinction of Deviant Sexual Interests." But in the spring of 1973, an Oakland-based group of social scientists, lawyers, and physicians formed a committee to prevent funding of the Violence Center by the state of California. The group, known as COPAP (Committee Opposing Psychiatric Abuse of Prisoners), grew out of opposition to the planned psychosurgical operations proposed earlier through the CCJ and the University of California. Two of COPAP's members, Dr. Lee Coleman and Ed Opton, were particularly vigorous in bringing about a critical reevaluation of the Violence Center. In April 1973, Dr. Coleman, a child psychiatrist, had this to say when he appeared before a Senate Committee on Health and Welfare: "This is not a proposal for any kind of scientific endeavor. I think this is essentially a political endeavor using a scientific and medical veneer." During his testimony, Dr. Coleman traced the state's interest in the Violence Center to "an underlying hidden agenda—the development of more sophisticated techniques for law enforcement." He warned against the Center's "using medicine and psychiatry as a veneer for techniques which could be used for law enforcement."

Three months later, COPAP, along with seven other plaintiffs, brought suit against the Center in order to block its million-dollar allocation for 1973–74. So far no decision has been reached regarding the Center's ultimate funding, but there are indications that funding for such a project is still a very real possibility. In a letter to me in January 1974, the chairman of the Health and Welfare Committee asked for "your opinion as to what guidelines or controls should be attached to such funding." Such an inquiry, in my mind, skirts the basic issue of the propriety of social and behavioral scientists collaborating with law enforcement agencies. I'm convinced that these collaborations are ominous for our personal freedoms. In the words of Lee Coleman: "These coalitions have mutual benefits: with newly acquired powers and prestige, researchers keep working and law enforcement is provided with control techniques fully legitimized by the stamp of scientific research."

"Man Against Man"

The prisons offer another recent example of collaboration between government and behavior technologists. The history of this collaboration involves such strange bedfellows as an expert on Korean brainwashing and a psychiatrist specializing in "attack therapy."

It all began in 1962 when the then director of the United States Bureau of Prisons, James V. Bennett, sponsored a symposium for social scientists and correctional administrators to explore the possibilities of future cooperative projects between the two groups. The papers were later published in *Corrective Psychiatry and Journal of Social Therapy*. One paper, "Man Against Man," by Professor Edgar Schein of the Massachusetts Institute of Technology, became the inspiration over the next decade for many prison administrators. In some respects it is the most influential document ever written on prison or management rehabilitation.

"In order to produce marked change of behavior and/or attitude, it is necessary to weaken, undermine, or remove the supports to the old patterns of behavior and the old attitudes," wrote Schein, and he suggested "breaking emotional ties by severing all contacts between the prisoner and those whom he cares about," and establishing instead a "total environment which inflexibly provides rewards and punishments only in terms of the new behavior and attitudes to be obtained."

Professor Schein's thesis derived from his study of the "brainwashing" methods used by the Chinese Communists on American prisoners of war. An expert on methods of indoctrination, Schein warned his listeners against too hasty a response to the idea of "brainwashing." "The model of behavior and attitude change is a general one which can encompass phenomena as widely separated as brainwashing and rehabilitation in a prison or mental hospital." Drawing from the Communists' successes in creating American turncoats, Schein suggested that the use "of the same techniques and the service of different goals . . . may be quite acceptable to us." Under the heading "Social Disorganization and the Creation of Mutual Distrust," Professor Schein set down the basic goals of the new "rehabilitation." "If one wants to produce behavior inconsistent with the person's standard of conduct, first disorganize the group which supports these standards, then undermine his other emotional supports, then put him into a new and ambiguous situation for which the standards are unclear and *then put pressure on him*." (Italics mine.)

In the last thirteen years Professor Schein's proposals have spearheaded many of the federal Bureau of Prisons' most ambitious prison projects. In her book *Kind and Usual Punishment,* Jessica Mitford cites a letter that was smuggled out of the federal penitentiary at Marion, Illinois, by the Federal Prisoners' Coalition, a special group of segregated prisoners who refused to participate in the behavioral-control programs. The letter discusses the "quiet beginning" in 1968 by the Department of Justice and the U.S. Bureau of Prisons to "determine firsthand how effective a weapon brainwashing might be for the U.S. Department of Justice's further use." It describes how the inmates' relations with families and friends were severed by their confinement in a prison perhaps halfway across the nation, isolation, deprivation of male personal belongings, dietary and severe exercise restrictions—all followed until the prisoner agreed to participate in the behavior-modification program. With acquiescence, the prisoner moved up the ladder of privilege, eventually coming into contact with a "prisoner thought reform team" where the real treatment began; "his emotional, behavioral and psychic characteristics are studied by the staff and prison paraprofessionals to detect vulnerable points of entry to stage attack sessions* around. During these sessions, on a progressively intensified basis, he is shouted at, his fears played on, his sensitivities ridiculed and concentrated efforts made to make him feel guilty for real or imagined characteristics of conduct. Every effort is made to heighten his suggestibility and weaken his character structure so that his emotional responses and thought flow will be brought under group and staff control as totally as possible."

A program built on these principles opened in September 1972, at the Bureau of Prisons' medical center in Springfield, Missouri. Named Project START (Special Treatment and Rehabilitation Training), the program "aimed to promote behavioral and attitudinal change in that element of the prison institutional population which has chronically demonstrated inability to affect adherence to established regulations." An involuntary program for prisoners "unable to adjust satisfac-

---

* Attack sessions are later to form the basis for Dr. Martin Groder's treatment program at Marion, Illinois (see page 43).

torily to a regular penal institution" and true to the methods of behavior modification, it involved a status system in which obedient prisoners received rewards of increased status and privilege. At Level 1, which lasted a minimum of three weeks, the prisoner remained in solitary confinement without mail or personal belongings. After the attainment of a perfect rating for cooperation and a satisfactory rating for such things as grooming and room neatness came Level 2, with its permission for limited commissary, library, and visiting privileges. After six months and another "perfect record" for cooperation, Level 3 followed, with opportunities for full-time work, increased visiting privileges, more money, greater access to the library, and so on.

Project START would still be cited as a "model" program if it were not for the efforts of two lawyers, Arpiar Saunders and Barbara Milstein, of the National Prison Project of the American Civil Liberties Union. From the beginning of the National Prison Project in July 1972, Saunders and Milstein had been in touch with prisoners in most of the larger prisons across the country. According to Ms. Milstein, a petite, attractive woman in her early thirties, the key source of information about Project START came from her correspondence with prisoners transferred to Springfield for assignment to the project. "From this we got a prisoner's eye view of what are the most oppressive issues to the largest number of prisoners. In this case it was Project START. So we went out to Springfield and helped some of the prisoners to file a writ of habeas corpus."

In January 1974 seven prisoners filed suit. They alleged: (1) that the compulsory transfer of prisoners to Project START violated the constitutional rights of due process and equal protection of the law; (2) that START constituted punishment and not treatment and that the prisoners had an absolute right to be transferred from the project without penalty; (3) that START violated the rights of freedom of speech, freedom of religion, freedom from unwarranted search and seizure, and freedom from invasion of privacy. "In a sense, Project START represented the very worst in new innovations in the prisons," Ms. Milstein told me. "Positive reinforcement was supposed to be used to help change behavior, but the prison guards weren't trained to observe and interpret behavior. Instead, they were accustomed to viewing behavior as either hostile or aggressive, and act accordingly."

In addition, prison classification systems added to the mutual frustration and antagonism between prisoners and the authorities. "If you wanted to keep some prisoner confined to Level 1, you just kept labeling his behavior as hostile. In essence, you wind up with a punitive program resulting from a terribly basic misunderstanding about what is going on: the guards thought Project START represented an opportunity to change prisoners; they in turn saw it as a phony effort to control them according to new rules."

In response to the suit, the presiding judge ordered three expert witnesses to evaluate the merits of Project START. Harold Cohen, chairman of the Committee to Evaluate START and head of the Institute for Behavioral Research in Silver Spring, Maryland, summed up the opinion of the experts: "It is a terrible project, in terms both of science and ethics: in fact a dismal failure." Cohen, a controversial figure in behavior therapy with deviant youths, voiced outrage at the primitive understanding of behavior principles shown by those who ran Project START. "For one thing, I found the physical space in the START Project to be as offensive and as visually destructive as the prison's other solitary confinement facilities. The program offered little or no opportunity for the kind of individuality required to convert the metal and steel barred facilities into a more humane living environment." Cohen thought the project should be abolished and replaced by a program that would have "client representation." Specifically, he joined with Saunders and Milstein in objecting to the non-voluntarism of Project START. "I believe that they, even as convicted men, should be shown and clearly informed of the value of program alternatives available to them—the individual should have the option to join the behavior modification program and given form consent to his involvement in it."

Within a week of the submission of Cohen's report, the Bureau of Prisons announced the discontinuance of Project START. Conspicuously avoiding any reference to the panel's report, Theodore Swift, assistant to the director of the Bureau, issued a statement that the decision to dismantle the program was "essentially an economic one" and warned against viewing the decision as an indication that the Prison Bureau was abandoning the concept of behavior modification.

Four months later, on July 31, 1974, a decision was reached regarding Project START. In a tersely worded opinion, U.S. District Judge John W. Oliver in Kansas City, Missouri, declared that the procedures for transferring prisoners into the START program were unconstitutional. And for the first time a legal opinion was expressed regarding the constitutional rights of prisoners to elect *not* to participate in programs designed to modify their behavior. According to Alvin J. Bronstein, executive director of the ACLU Prison Project, "The decision is of great importance in that it recognizes that any attempt to experimentally change a person's mind and behavior is a very serious matter." The response of the U.S. Bureau of Prisons to the case was different. As Theodore Swift said: "We've got to seek other ways to try to reach those persons. We have a moral obligation to do something."

What other ways may be in preparation was not entirely clear. Certainly the Bureau of Prisons is committed to at least one more major "innovative" program using behavior modification. In 1974 a behavioral research center was scheduled to open in Butner, North Carolina, on forty-three acres of land described as a "mud flat." Originally named the U.S. Behavioral Research Center, the government's newest prison has already been renamed in response to mounting criticism: it is now called the Federal Center for Correction Research.

The warden of the new facility is Dr. Martin Groder, a thirty-four-year-old psychiatrist with previous prison experience at the federal penitentiary at Marion, Illinois. Dr. Groder is most renowned for his development while at Marion of a treatment known as Asklepieion therapy or more pointedly, "attack therapy"—in essence, a remodeled version of Dr. Schein's techniques of the 1960s. Dr. Groder arrived at his unique treatment method by combining transactional analysis with Synanon attack therapy designed to cure drug addicts. During his residency at the Langley-Porter Neuropsychiatric

Institute in San Francisco, Dr. Groder came into contact with Eric Berne, author of *Games People Play*. From Berne he learned the transactional-analysis approach of dividing the ego into three states: parent, child, and adult. In the parental ego state, participants "are barred from parental figures and reproduce the feelings, attitudes, behavior and responses of these figures." The child's ego state reproduces the individual's behavior as a child. Finally, in the adult ego state, behavior is based on "the rational calculation of probabilities derived from objectively gathered data." Treatment consists in the participants' becoming aware of their responses in terms of parent, child, or adult ego states and then, with the assistance of a therapist, beginning to analyze their own behavior for the purpose of encouraging the adult ego state.

During Dr. Groder's first assignment as warden at Marion, he discovered that transactional analysis alone was not effective with some of the prisoners; they faked participation and ridiculed those involved in transactional analysis. Dr. Groder referred to this as "making fools of," a term he uses in a technical sense, and set out to overcome it by introducing Synanon attack therapy. Here is his description of that attack therapy in action: "Eight of them walked into the room and sat down—and I proceeded to rip them off, one after the other. I just shit all over them about all the things that had come to my attention that were so obvious to me about the trickiness, the lies, the misrepresentations—their aimed dedication to stupidity—the whole ball of dirty wax." In Groder's words these sessions were "very traumatic to the men," who were encouraged to abuse certain prisoners verbally in an effort to change their behavior. Traumatic also because "the men couldn't believe their good, friendly old Jewish psychiatrist was doing this to them." In addition, he says, "They were defenseless because of the incredible lies they were living."

At the end of one attack session in November 1969, a group member was stabbed to death as a result of a homosexual jealousy fantasy that had been mobilized during the intensive Asklepieion session. In response to this, Groder's unit at Marion was closed for a month by the prison authorities and, in his words, "because of an instigating homosexual this event, external to the program, almost terminated the program." By 1970 Dr. Groder reopened his unit and formed the Asklepieion Society, composed of graduates trained to conduct attack therapy sessions on their own. Each trainee was charged with spreading his philosophy of "the winner" throughout the prison system. "The winner," Dr. Groder has written, "no longer blames others, his parents, the police, his wife, bad luck, or the *prison system*—for who he is."

At Butner, Dr. Groder's attack therapy will be combined with primal-scream therapy, and inmates "will be able to regress and relive and abreact traumas of various kinds from childhood." In a behavior research section composed of 340 men, efforts will be made "to improve prisoner rehabilitation programs" by another try at transactional analysis combined with Asklepieion and a new program of yoga.

A prominent consideration in the structure of Dr. Groder's unit will be obtaining informed consent. Where Project START was entirely compulsory, Dr. Groder is committed to accepting "volunteer inmates" who will enter the program only after giving informed consent. But this issue of informed consent in prisons is a knotty one. "Informed consent is simply impossible in a prison situation which is by nature inherently coercive," Ms. Milstein has said. In a formal statement the ACLU Prison Project has demanded "the immediate termination of all ongoing and planned medical experimentation and behavior-modification programs of the Department of Justice and Public Welfare." Once again the issue of informed consent forms the basis for a sweeping condemnation of prison research on behavior modification: "It is our position that as long as the prison environment remains inherently coercive, no set of regulations will be sufficient to insure truly informed consent." The Prison Project cites the recent Michigan court case forbidding psychosurgery on a prisoner as supportive of its position. "Accumulation of substantial doubts about the validity of the various components of consent leads to the holding that there cannot be legally adequate consent."

Indications suggest that the battlelines are now being

drawn between civil libertarians and the supporters of the Bureau of Prisons' behavior-modification programs. One recent clash has come over the Contingency Management Program funded by the LEAA in Virginia. Like Project START, it is located in a maximum-security prison, the Virginia state penitentiary, and consists of several "stages" that the prisoner must attain to earn increasingly liberal prison privileges. By the time the prisoner has reached the final stage, Stage 4, he is actively involved in vocational-guidance courses in a minimum-security setting in a neighboring prison. The transition, however, is a lot more than geographic. To get to Stage 4 the prisoner must earn "points," which are awarded for such things as neatness, making his own bed, engaging in "polite" conversation free of profanity or abuse. So far, twelve inmates have graduated to lower-security prisons while participating in the CMP. "These were real troublemakers; today they're gentlemen," states E. Scott Geller, one of the psychologists who designed the program. The response of the ACLU, however, has been less enthusiastic; lawyers there have threatened suit if the program is not discontinued. "Dr. Geller seems to have an idealistic notion that his program is going to make prisoners better people," says Thomas Howard of the ACLU. "All he's doing is helping the prison to make them more docile."

The implications of all of this for prisons are of course profound. If the prisons continue to function as they have in the past, and if they are ultimately forbidden to incorporate new techniques such as those suggested by Dr. Groder, the end result may be a return to narrowly conceived punitive activities rather than the rehabilitative measures that have taken so many years to achieve. To Barbara Milstein this may even be tolerable if, ultimately, the prison authorities realize that the prison *system* and not the prisoners are at fault. "As long as our prisons remain large warehouse institutions, it is impossible to test any program and determine its validity." In the long run, Ms. Milstein and her associates are holding out for a different prison system. "We have to get beyond the idea that community protection is only a matter of barbed wires and high walls. As long as that view prevails, behavior modification of any sort cannot work and can only give the same results no matter what behavioral technology is brought to bear. As long as you have the same environment you will have the same results."

In early 1975 Dr. Martin Groder resigned from the Bureau of Prisons following a reassignment to the medical center for Federal Prisons at Springfield, Missouri. In response to Groder's parting charges that the Bureau of Prisons is re-adopting a "warehousing" approach to prisoners, Norman Carlson, Director of the Federal Bureau of Prisons, stated: "The Bureau facility will not necessarily take any or all or a large part of what Groder developed."

Behavior Control: An X-Rated Science

Behavior control is rapidly becoming the most compelling bioethical issue facing our society. Psychosurgery, behavior modification among prisoners and the institutionalized, government-supported research on violence—all these efforts are turning out in the final analysis to be subtle and scientifically respectable ways of avoiding necessary changes in our society. In the case of prisons, for example, some people would have us believe that the fault lies not in the prisons but in the prisoners whose "behavior" must somehow be "controlled." Never mind the present truths about prisons, with their 75 per cent recidivism rate; never mind the $1.5 billion dollars a year spent on corrections; never mind that our elaborate prison facilities haven't worked. The answer must be more of the same: larger prisons, increased isolation of prisoners from the community, increasingly pernicious intrusion into other people's minds. Predictively, this will lead to further spiraling of the process of dehumanization and the need for even more "behavior control."

A similar course is being followed with regard to violence in our society. In response to escalating levels of violence, particularly in our nation's largest cities, people like Drs. West, Ervin, Sweet, and Mark seem to believe that the problems reside inside the brains of the violently predisposed. They are content to ignore, or relegate to only circumstantial importance, the social realities that lead to this vicious cycle of social deprivation, frustration, and further violence. Such an attitude results, not surprisingly, in the wrong question being posed. Instead of, "What we can do *for* the violent person?" we ask, "What can we do *to* the violent person?"

A radically altered course of action is called for. Continuance of the present search for sophisticated biotechnological "controls" of behavior can lead only to more dehumanization. Rather than emphasizing the control of behavior, we must concentrate on the reason why more and more of us are coming under the purview of behavior controllers. As I have tried to make plain, a much larger issue is at stake than psychosurgery or behavior modification in prisons or government agencies. To focus on these narrower issues is to blind ourselves to the larger social realities that have created a desire for "behavior control" in the first place. As a neurologist, I am convinced that psychosurgery, for instance, can be helpful in certain uncommon but highly specific diseases. Those who would outlaw psychosurgery altogether are as unreasonable and repressive as those who expect it to solve all our social problems. Psychosurgery *may* have some limited medical psychiatric uses. It should *never* be used in the service of social control. Of much more critical importance than these specific issues, however, is the increasingly prevalent view that biotechnology is an appropriate method of tackling complex and multidetermined social problems. Succinylcholine at Atascadero; the LEAA funding for the Center for Prevention of Violence; Butner; Project START; covert sensitization; Dr. Orlando Andy's operations on "hyperactive children"—behind all these bizarre activities lies an article of faith that has been accepted without being examined: that biotechnologists can provide us with the solutions to *social problems*.

Take "hyperactive children," for example. If a kid can't sit still in the classroom, behavioral-control technologists would have us drug him into a semistupor. If this doesn't work, shove a stereotactic probe into his amygdala. But don't look into his classroom; don't observe the repressiveness of his teacher; don't investigate the chilling impersonality of his parents—focus instead on the nonconforming kid, and somehow change him. It is attitudes such as these that must change.

I believe the fundamental bioethical imperative for behavioral scientists today is to have the courage to renounce all collaboration with forces seeking to "control" or "modify" or "engineer" human responses. In a country of limited economic opportunity for the vast majority of men and women, whose behavior should be "controlled"? Until practical means are available to assuage human grief and trouble, by what right can behavior scientists assist in "controlling" the free expression of certain kinds of behavior, just because that behavior is perceived as a threat by those wielding power? In a very real sense, "behavior control" is an ethically indefensible and scientifically spurious pursuit, given our present social realities. In a word it is *obscene*.

Under the rubric of "research," behavioral scientists today are contributing their specialized knowledge to the government in order that it can develop increasingly sophisticated tools of repression. This is possible largely because of the widespread and traditional misconception that scientists operate outside the usual social and political frames of reference. Nothing can be further from the truth. When psychosurgery in prisons is paid for by the government and studies on prison reform are not, this decision is ideological, not scientific. Unfortunately, until recently, such decisions have failed to stimulate the confrontations demanded of social and ideological doctrines in the making.

But behavior control is only one aspect of the emerging new biotechnology. I have been struck with a generally uncritical acceptance by many scientists, men of diverse training and interest, of the idea that they have a mission to produce the "hardware" necessary to sustain the social status quo.

To them, it is appropriate to develop new methods of behavior "control" and ignore the possibility that "disruptive" or "disturbed" behavior may often be the stimulus for necessary social change. For these reasons I have become convinced that decisions regarding the control and future directions of biotechnology must be taken out of the hands of the "experts" and instead be debated publicly within the context of politics and ideology, where they rightfully belong. One area in which this clearly must be done is in the expanding application of what has come to be called "genetic engineering." Those who would control our behavior are no less interested in manipulating our genes.

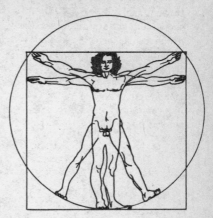

Part Two

Genetic Engineering: Opportunity or Trap?

Wombs for Hire

It's 10:00 P.M. We're in a small operating room in a hospital two hours from London. The patient, a twenty-six-year-old woman, has just been given an anesthetic. All is in readiness for a most unusual and controversial operation.

The surgeon, Patrick C. Steptoe, makes his incision, a small one below the navel, only large enough to enable the insertion of a tiny manipulating forceps. With this he grasps the ovaries, the egg-producing organs located on both sides of the uterus. By means of a special suction apparatus he removes as many of the tiny eggs as he can find, perhaps fifteen or sixteen. The eggs are then transferred to a small dish containing a special mix of nutrients that has been worked out over many years of painstaking research.

Dr. Robert G. Edwards of the Cambridge University Physiology Laboratory is waiting on the other side of the operating rooms. He receives the specimen, identifies the eggs, and washes them with another solution prior to placing them in a suspension of sperm. Dr. Edwards' special skill involves identifying preovulatory oocytes—those eggs at precisely the right stage of development for fertilization. Then the eggs and sperm are brought into contact in a special medium where they are exposed to a flow of gas of specific composition and concentration (this part of the laboratory, as well as the operating section, is sterile; the slightest contamination, even by ordinarily harmless organisms, will sabotage the incubation).

At intervals, the culture media are removed and studied under a microscope for evidence of fertilization—the union of the egg with one of the fifty thousand or so sperm in each tiny drop of suspension previously placed in the culture media. At a certain point a doubling of the number of pronuclei in the center of the new cell signals that fertilization has taken place. The new embryo is then placed in another medium and is observed periodically for cell division. At the sixteen- and thirty-two-cell stage, about four days later, the most delicate part of the procedure begins.

The patient is returned to the operating room, this time fully awake. The embryo is picked up under microscopic control and introduced into the cervix, the entry zone leading into the uterus. The patient is then taken to her room to await evidence of the success or failure of the operation. Over the next few weeks sex hormones will be monitored for evidence of pregnancy. If successful, a previously sterile woman will be able to carry a child fertilized entirely outside her body.

"We first became interested in embryo transfers as a means of helping those women who cannot have children because of deformities or abnormalities in their oviducts," Dr. Steptoe explained. In the United States somewhere between 12 and 15 per cent of couples are not able to have children because of an infertility problem. A considerable number of these marriages are childless because of defects in the woman's fallopian tubes, the path from the ovary to the womb. The most frequent cause of infertility is blockage of these fallopian tubes, resulting in a "hangup" of the newly fertilized egg. On rare occasions the egg goes on to mature within the tube, a dangerous occurrence because of the potential for the rupture of the tube and its contained blood vessels. But the usual result of blocked fallopian tubes is the death of the fertilized egg and a permanent frustrating and usually anguishing sterility. The Steptoe-Edwards procedure would bypass the fallopian tubes by artificially maintaining the newly fertilized egg through the stages that it would normally undergo during its passage through the fallopian tube and into the uterus.

The embryo-transfer technique raises the possibility of influencing the process of reproduction in a more direct way than most scientists ever thought possible. One application involves the identification of various forms of chromosome-induced deformity. Spontaneous abortions frequently result from defects in the chromosomes, the genetic material responsible for inheritance. Detailed studies on the chromosomes of artificially fertilized embryos promise to supply data on various forms of deformity.

With increasing maternal age the incidence of deformity in the offspring increases. Mongolism, for instance, is principally seen in the children of mothers over thirty-five years of age. Mongolism can also result when the time of implantation is delayed. The question is, How long a delay is sufficient to produce a mongol? So far there has been no way of finding out. Such data might be obtained from the embryo-transfer technique by deliberately delaying fertilization in the artificial media.

Another potential benefit involves evaluation of the effects of drugs and X rays on the early stages of human development. Agreement already exists that drugs and X rays are teratogenic—literally, monster producing—in the growing fetus. But critical questions remain: How much radiation? What drugs and in what doses? Answers might be found via the Steptoe-Edwards route where the organism could be recovered by abortion at any stage and compared with other fetuses aborted earlier or later in the laboratory-initiated pregnancy.

With the embryo technique, early preimplantation embryos (up to about the eight- or sixteen-cell stage, where implantation in the uterus usually takes place) may be typed for deformities or abnormalities. This has been done for years in experimental animals by a simple technique. First, a small piece of tissue—even just a few cells—is removed from the early embryo and grown in a culture medium. If abnormalities are detected in the resulting tissue culture grown from the extracted cells, the embryo can be aborted, thus eliminating the birth of a defective. This seems a feasible procedure in humans as well, since animal experiments have demonstrated that embryos can tolerate a considerable amount of manipulation without harm (this does not hold after implantation, when specific organs such as the heart and brain are developing; even slight interference at this stage can cause deformities and spontaneous abortion).

As a future refinement in complexity, embryos may be stored frozen while the growth of the extracted cell colonies is awaited. If everything is proceeding according to schedule, the embryo can then be unfrozen and implanted within the uterus. This was accomplished with cattle embryos in 1974 at the Agricultural Research Council's Unit of Reproductive Physiology and Biochemistry at Cambridge University. Normal cows were artificially inseminated; on the tenth day of pregnancy, the eggs were removed and frozen; six days later, they were slowly thawed out and transplanted into the uterus of another cow. Of twenty-two eggs thus frozen, only two were successfully implanted; and one bull, Frosty, was actually born: the first large mammal born from a deep-frozen embryo. So far it is not technically possible to freeze fertilized human ova, but this is promised in the next few years. "The difficulties should not be underrated, but they are not insuperable," according to Dr. Edwards.

Another beneficial spin-off from the embryo-transfer technique concerns sex-linked diseases. It has been known for centuries that certain diseases appear only in males. Hemophilia is a classic example; its tendency to uncontrolled bleeding due to a blood defect in the clotting mechanism leads to difficulty in controlling hemorrhage, even after minor injuries. Hemophilia is transmitted from the mother but affects only her sons; her daughters will be carriers for the disease and, like the mother, transmit it only to sons. If the male sex chromosome, known as the Y chromosome, was identified in the early embryonic state, a potentially crippling disease could be avoided by selecting only embryos of the female sex for placement in the mother's womb.

More theoretical is the use of the embryo-transfer technique to treat abnormalities detected soon after fertilization. There were early indications that such treatment would one day be possible. In 1966 Dr. Beatrice Mintz of the Institute for Cancer Research in Philadelphia performed a now famous experiment which demonstrated the newly fertilized egg's capacity to withstand profound modifications in its structure. Dr. Mintz removed the fertilized eggs from two pregnant mice, one black mouse and one white one. She then treated these eggs with enzymes which dissolved part of the protecting coat surrounding the eggs, thus enabling them to be recombined into a single growing organism made up of the cell lines from the white and the black mice. The mice born after this procedure demonstrated extensive pigmentation of the coat and skin of the tail. Instead of a white mouse or a black mouse, Dr. Mintz wound up with a mixture of both, known as a chimera: the partial expression of two independent cell lines. By a cruel trick of nature, a similar result was later observed in a black woman who gave birth to a "zebra child" with alternating bands of white and black skin on the body surface. It has been thought that this resulted from an extremely rare event: the fusion of two independently growing eggs resulting from two fertilizations, one with the sperm from a Caucasian, the other with the sperm from a black. Both Dr. Mintz's experimental work and the unfortunate "zebra child" demonstrated that, under certain conditions and shortly after fertilization, eggs could be fused. This raised an even more intriguing question: could other substances such as viruses be introduced into the egg in its early growth stages?

The name for this process of injecting new cells into the early fertilized ova for the correction of disease is known as gene therapy. It too bears on the Steptoe-Edwards embryo-transfer technique. Theoretically—and all is theory at this point, since deliberate and controlled alterations of the genes are not possible even in animals—a defect in the culture cells would be corrected *in vitro* by the insertion of a virus; then the cured cells would be replaced in a developing organism by self-replication. Ideally the treated cells would grow preferentially and determine the biologic fate of the organism. The application of this work to humans involves, first, the identification of the embryo at risk for deformity, and second, control of the effects of the donated cells on the other normal aspects of development. So far the problem hasn't been worked out in humans. There have been demonstrations, however, of the abilities of viruses to attach themselves to living cells and bring about biochemical changes. The Shope virus, for instance, carries the information for the synthesis of a special enzyme, arginase, which breaks down the amino acid arginine. It has been known for years that rabbits infected with the virus retain a low blood-arginine level. When the virus is injected into mice, rats, or monkeys, their blood-arginine levels are also observed to fall. All of which has caused scientists to speculate: "What is the effect of the virus on the animal handlers and scientists who have worked with the virus-infected rabbits?"

To find out, Dr. Stanfield Rogers of the Oak Ridge National Laboratory in Oak Ridge, Tennessee, studied the blood-arginine levels of those occupationally exposed to the Shope virus. Over half of them showed a low blood-arginine level in the absence of any detectable symptoms. Dr. Rogers next turned his attention to the life span of the virus within living cells. He found that one laboratory worker who had not worked with the virus for twenty years still retained a low blood-arginine level. Another, who had deliberately inoculated himself with the virus thirty years previously, had a normal circulating blood-arginine level when checked by Dr. Rogers, which suggested that the virus had lost potency over time. Does this data mean that the Shope virus has a lifetime within the body cells of twenty years and would die out after thirty years? Probably not. More likely the differing results on the virus's life span indicate that presently unknown factors influence the propagation of viruses within body cells.

The application of this type of research goes something like this: First, the identification of an embryo with a deficient ability to break down arginine. In its fully developed form this disease, argininemia, is manifested by severe mental retardation, epilepsy, and other metabolic problems. Second, the early introduction of the passenger virus carrying the information for arginase formation. This process, known as gene insertion, has the potential for curing incurable diseases like argininemia. Unfortunately, it also has the potential for spreading unfavorable genetic capacities such as cancer-inducing viruses and viruses capable of inducing antibiotic-resistant bacteria. So critical has the issue become, and so unprepared are we for the potential hazards of this type of research, that a special National Academy of Science committee recommended a moratorium in July 1974 on gene-insertion experiments. As this book was going to press, scientists continued to debate whether or not to comply with this call for a self-imposed moratorium on research, the first such effort in the history of science.

One final application of embryo transfer is nuclear cloning—the most dramatic and publicized aspect of all. In

1958 Professor J. B. Gurdon demonstrated that, in frogs, each body cell has a full complement of genetic material which can give rise to a complete replica of the original frog. Dr. Gurdon showed that it was possible to transplant the nuclei from cells lying in the toad's gut into another frog's ova from which the nuclear material had been removed. The resulting toad had the identical genetic characteristics of the donor toad. Each living cell, whether from the skin, the liver, or the brain—in fact, from any organ in the body—presumably contains the complete genetic makeup of the organism. Previously it was considered that brain cells and liver cells, for instance, were derived from completely different cell lines. Dr. Gurdon's work suggested that somewhere along the line of development brain and liver cells become specialized to perform certain functions but still maintain the basic genetic cloning for the potential replication of a whole organism. Most scientists believe that a similar situation exists in man: any cell in the body has the potential for duplicating a complete person.

The operative word here is *potential*. So far, cloning has been limited to aquatic frogs and has never been carried out in any mammal, least of all man. "Cloning is a flight of the imagination," according to Dr. Steptoe. "There is absolutely no evidence to show that it can be done in mammals." Dr. Edwards is in complete agreement with this. "It might be feasible, but all the results so far show that when the nucleus is taken from an adult cell and is placed in an egg, many of the offspring will die. It now seems doubtful that the transferred nucleus is incorporated into the embryo."

Further doubts about the possibility of human cloning have been raised by the studies of the effect of the interuterine environment on the resulting organism. In 1958 an embryologist named Dr. Ann McLaren, at the university of Edinburgh, performed an embryo-transfer experiment on mice with five lumbar vertebrae in their spinal canal. She implanted the embryos from a mother with five vertebrae into a foster mother who had six vertebrae. The result? "The newborn mice all were found to resemble their foster and not their true mother." A larger conclusion one might draw from this is that the embryo is strongly affected by changes within the womb. Would a cloned child then necessarily have the same attributes as the donor?

Dr. Edwards has gone on record as a disbeliever in the imminence of cloning. "We conclude that this method—which has been greatly overwritten as an immediate possibility—requires a great deal of proving before it can be considered a practical means of conserving genetically superior individuals."

In an attempt to resolve some conflicting views on embryo transfer, I spoke with Patrick Steptoe in his laboratory in Oldham General Hospital, near Manchester, England. A nattily dressed, precise man somewhere in his late fifties, Dr. Steptoe explained his personal reasons for continuing with the embryo-transfer work:

"One of the hardest and heartrending aspects of a gynecologist's practice involves trying to help women who want to have children but who are most certainly permanently sterile," he said. "One can't be one hundred per cent sure, of course, that sterility is absolute as long as ovaries, oviducts, and a uterus are present. Still, after some years of experience you learn to recognize those women who, short of a miracle, are never going to conceive. I've seen the misery that these people endure, and it's not just a wife and her husband. It affects so many others: parents, relatives, one's relationship with neighbors and friends, and so on. Now with increasing liberal abortion laws, the possibility of adoption is becoming less and less of an option. But with the further development and refinement of embryo transfer we are going to be able to help some of these people."

The demand for embryo transfer has been increasing, ironically enough, at a time when funds for transfer research have almost disappeared. But a steady stream of patients remains in contact with Steptoe and awaits the perfection of this transfer technique.

"One of my patients is particularly pathetic in her desire for a child," he told me. "She is a nurse with a better than average understanding of some of the problems involved. She was born without a uterus but has functioning ovaries.

I've proved by surgical examination of the eggs that they are normal and if fertilized a child could develop. In the absence of a uterus, of course, this is impossible. This unfortunate woman has a sister who has offered to have a fertilized egg implanted in her own uterus. This way the mother and father will be the natural ones, but the biological mother in terms of carrying the child through a pregnancy will be the aunt. I'm fully aware, of course, that there is no precedent for this kind of thing."

Within months of my conversation with Dr. Patrick Steptoe, Dr. Douglas Bevis, who twenty years previously had made the first systematic attempt to sample amniotic fluid, announced that three "test-tube babies" had been born and were developing normally. That same week came the results of a National Academy of Science panel on the assessment of biotechnology. The report, written in September 1972 and suppressed because of disagreements between the panel and a review committee regarding its publication, predicted that a successful embryo transfer would be carried out within two years. More important than its predictive value, however, is the light the report sheds on the conflicts likely to be stimulated by a successful embryo transfer. Consider three possible transfer situations:

In the first and simplest situation a husband and wife who are unable to have their own child because of fallopian-tube disease elect to have a child by *in vitro* fertilization and embryo transfer. The beneficial results are obvious. Many potentially successful parents who are now frustrated in their desire for a child would have available to them a new technique that, if all goes well, would provide them with a healthy normal child, *their own child.* The key qualifier here is "if all goes well." Animal experiments with mice have already demonstrated a low overall success rate of about one live mouse for every twenty-five eggs exposed to fertilization. A similar situation may be found in humans. Several laparoscopies may be required for the mother, as well as repeated implantations, before a successful transfer could be achieved.

What are the chances for malformation? At this point nobody knows. Prospective "transfer parents" would have to accept the scientists' inability to guarantee them a healthy child. Further, if a severely deformed child resulted from the procedure, no precedent exists for what should be done with it. Can the parents ask that it be destroyed? Should they? Would they? Would the operating surgeon have any liability in such a case? Would he have any responsibility to ease the parents' dilemma by destroying the child himself when a severe malformation became obvious? These are just some of the questions concerned with the *physical* aspects of embryo transfer. (Consider also a few of the psychological consequences of "test-tube babies." As a member of the group of children conceived by technology, a test-tube child and its parents would be faced with conflicting demands for privacy on the one hand and a predictable demand from various scientific sources for information on the child's development.)

Consider too a second application of the new technique: the "adopted" embryo. Here the embryo transferred after laboratory fertilization is from a stranger. Either an anonymous or known female donor provides the egg; the husband or another donor provides the sperm. One use of such a procedure would be for women with absent or diseased ovaries. Along with the previously mentioned problems, the "adopted" embryo transfer introduces the knotty question of the mother's identity. Who is the *real* mother? Is she the one who provides the egg for fertilization or the one who carries the child through the nine months of development within the uterus? In the case where the "donor mother" is known, she may retain more of an interest in the child than the "carrier mother" may tolerate. Where the "mothers" are related, the conflict may grow even more intense. One example of the type of problem that might arise would be a possible dispute when the "donor mother" changed her mind after the implantation and wanted the embryo from "her egg" aborted.

The third transfer situation is the most controversial of all: the transfer of an embryo into the womb of a "paid" recipient. In most cases the father and mother would provide the egg and sperm but for various reasons would elect to have another woman carry it to term. One might imagine such a situation among women with pathological fears of pregnancy or those with a history of repeated miscarriages caused by subtle biochemical abnormalities in their uterus. One could even imagine an industry built around a concept of "wombs for hire," an industry with potentially disastrous consequences. For one thing, the "identity crisis" of a child born from such a procedure could be unresolvable. Based on studies of the fantasies of adopted children, we could expect obsessions and preoccupations such as, "Who loved the child more—the 'mother' who provided half of the child's genetic makeup, or the 'mother' who made the child's independent existence possible?"

Many scientists think such questions too speculative, almost irrelevant to the issue of developing the embryo-transfer technique. They cite the professional ethics of the operating surgeon as a protection from such things. "I think this 'wombs for hire' stuff is all a lot of nonsense," Dr. Steptoe told me. "I can't imagine any ethical gynecologist implanting a fertilized egg into a surrogate mother just on the whim of a natural mother who didn't want to go through a pregnancy." But other scientists are less convinced that "wombs for hire" is mere "nonsense." They fear embryo transfer is a paradigm of biologic technology out of control. In one respect they are certainly correct: a good bit more is at stake in the embryo-transfer work than the humanitarian principle of helping childless couples to have children. Dr. McLaren put it succinctly: "If we decide that egg-transfer techniques are available and have some clinical usefulness, we must accept the corollary that development will not stop at the management of the subfertile woman."

A particularly vocal critic of the embryo-transfer work is Dr. Leon Kass of the Kennedy Institute and principal author of the National Academy of Science panel on the assessment of biotechnology. Physician-biochemist-philosopher, Dr. Kass was among the first to warn of the potential bioethical hazards of the embryo-transfer work. In addition, while others seemed uncertain of a stance to take in this rapidly expanding field, Dr. Kass has come down hard against "test-tube babies."

"What is new about embryo transfer is a divorce of the generation of new life from human sexuality and ultimately from the confines of the human body. Sexual intercourse will no longer be needed for generating new life. This novelty leads to two others: there is a new co-progenitor, the embryologist-geneticist-physician; and there is a new home for generation, the laboratory. The mysterious and intimate processes of generation are to be moved from the darkness of the womb to the bright (fluorescent) light of the laboratory."

If anything is more startling about Dr. Kass than his grasp of the issues it is probably his youth. While most bio-ethicists are well into their forties or fifties, Kass is a youthful thirty-five. Conservatively dressed, with a narrow tie and horn-rimmed glasses, he looks exactly as you would expect a scholar whose career began at the age of fifteen as a science major at the University of Chicago. What you don't expect—and I had never before encountered—is his combination of a physician and scientist's understanding of biotechnology with a philosopher's capacity to conjure up where that technology may be taking us.

To Dr. Kass, one of the most striking issues regarding embryo transfer is a purely technical one: the possibility of individual abnormalities developing as a result of the manipulation. "It's all very well to say that animal experiments have indicated a great resiliency against deformities in the implanted embryo, but so far we have absolutely no proof that the same situation will exist in man. There is at present no way of finding out whether or not the procedure of *in vitro* fertilization, culture, and transfer of human embryos will result in congenital anomalies, sterility, or mental retardation."

Once this uncertainty in the method is recognized, Dr. Kass slyly introduces the oldest injunction in all of medicine: *Primum non nocere*—do no harm. "There is a powerful moral objection to the implantation experiments. It does not rest upon arguments about the will of God or about natural rights. Instead, it rests upon that minimal principle of medical practice: do no harm. In these prospective experiments upon the newborn, it is not enough not to know of any grave defects: one needs to know with some confidence that there will be no such defects—or at least no more than there are without the procedure."

If there are risks involved in a medical procedure, then the patient must be apprised of the risk and must consent to it. With an embryo developing by a new and untested method, embryo transfer, appraisal of the risk is obviously impossible. This places these experiments, according to Dr. Kass, in the class of unethical experiments upon human subjects. He quoted the theologian Paul Ramsey: "The decisive moral verdict must be that we cannot rightfully get to know how to do this without conducting unethical experiments upon the unborn who must be the mishap (the dead and retarded ones) through whom we learn how."

Dr. Kass is also concerned about the ownership of the eggs removed for embryo transfer: Do and should these women know what is going to be done with their eggs? The Steptoe-Edwards procedure involves the prior administration of sex hormones to bring about multiple ovulation (superovulation) rather than the usual single monthly ovulation. This results in fifteen or sixteen eggs, only one of which can be chosen for implantation. "What happens to the other eggs?" asks Dr. Kass. "Would they ever be used in future embryo transfers, on another woman, for instance, whose eggs turned out to be less than optimum? Or are they discarded? If so, this is a distinctly different situation than prevails in abortion. The embryos discarded here are wanted, at least for a while. They are deliberately created, used for a time, and then deliberately destroyed. I am concerned about the effects and the attitude toward and respect for human life engendered in persons engaged in these practices. Who decides the ground for discards? What if there were another recipient available who wished to have an otherwise unwanted embryo? Shall we leave it so that discarding laboratory-grown embryos is a matter solely between a doctor and his plumber?"

Dr. Kass also wonders what the limits of the embryo-transfer use will be or even should be. "Why stop at couples? What about single women, widows, or lesbians? Adoption agencies now permit these women to adopt. Are they likely to be denied a chance to bear and deliver? But a decisive objection to the use of these techniques is that it requires and fosters both in thought and in deed exploitation of women and their bodies. And this just at a time when we're finally moving away from the sexual depersonalization of women."

Clearly, embryo transfer is calling for a rethinking of our concepts of sexuality, individual identity, and the outer limits of responsibility for the physical and mental health of our children. But even these considerations ignore what I think is the most important implication of embryo transfer: concentration of power by scientists in areas far removed from strictly scientific considerations. The history of the development of embryo transfers is a good example of this. Until recently, not much could be done about infertility. With improved surgical techniques, however, the repair of obstructed fallopian tubes became possible. In a sense we could say that this was a new power of "mankind"; but actually it was not so much a shared power as a power for a small group, in this case the operating surgeons. And, as often happens, a benefit exacts a cost. In this case the cost of the new power is our dependence on the biomedical technologists who are able to do this kind of surgery. With the development of embryo transfer the power involved has made a quantum jump; it involves no less than the act of creation itself. Embryo transfer is an unprecedented concentration of power in the hands of biomedical specialists who, in the exercise of that power, have so far operated without social restraint. But embryo transfer would not even be thinkable without an earlier venture into the manipulation and control of our reproduction: artificial insemination by a donor.

The Genetics of Anonymity

In 1971 seven women living in southern California became pregnant as a result of insemination with deep-frozen sperm from their husbands in Vietnam. The children born from this procedure, all of them healthy today, are part of an ever enlarging group whose numbers remain unknown. There is no registry of artificial insemination by donors (AID), as this procedure has come to be called, anywhere in the world; thus any computation of the extent of AID is only guesswork. But there is reason to believe that the procedure is increasing in popularity.

The concept of artificial insemination has a long history. As far back as 1776 an Italian scientist, L. Spallanzani, described the successful artificial insemination of a dog. No record exists of attempts at human artificial insemination, however, until the end of the eighteenth century when the physician John Hunter introduced the procedure. Hunter's technique is a simple one. Sperm is obtained by masturbation and deposited by means of a syringe in or near the cervix, the opening to the interior of the uterus. Since the life span of the sperm is limited, the timing of the insemination is critical. Every attempt is made to time this with ovulation, when the egg is released from the ovary. Since no certain method exists for determining this exactly in human beings, indirect measures are used today, such as watching for a small rise in the woman's body temperature or examining the cells from the vagina or checking the concentration of sex hormones in the woman's blood and urine. By these indirect measurements a success rate of 70 to 75 per cent has been achieved by some obstetricians over three or four months of attempted artificial insemination.

One of the early fears concerning the technique was the potential for the development of defective children. Studies over the last twenty years have proved that the technique is no more risky than routine pregnancy. The first indication of its relative harmlessness came from experiences in the breeding of cattle where, far from a rare procedure, artificial insemination has long been an accepted and successful technique aimed at improving the breed. By the late 1950s the ten millionth cow bred by artificial insemination occasioned a banquet by the milk marketing board in England. By 1970 artificial insemination represented over 60 per cent of all cattle breedings, with almost 3 million cows a year undergoing artificial insemination. The practice obviously would never have advanced as it did if abnormalities or defects had resulted from the procedure.

The experience in humans has been similarly favorable. In 1968 a study in *International Journal of Fertility* entitled "Physical and Mental Development of Children Born Following Artificial Insemination" reported on fifty-four AID children. The physical and mental development of these children was found to be "no way inferior to a similar controlled series." By 1957 one authority estimated that one hundred thousand babies had already been born in the United States since AID began. By 1966 another authority quoted a figure of ten thousand births by means of AID for that year alone. Contributing to this exponential increase was the development of the deep-frozen technique.

In 1866 Mantegazza formulated the concept of storing human sperm by freezing. Not until 1949 did technology catch up with the theory, when the chemical glycerol was discovered to have a protective effect on sperm placed in freezing conditions. For the first time the means were available to make practical Mantegazza's concept of storing sperm for future use. In 1952 came the first successful human pregnancy resulting from the use of frozen sperm. The deep-frozen technique was perfected in 1963 by the introduction of liquid nitrogen as a medium for freezing sperm. In 1973 Dr. Jerome Sherman reported that over five hundred normal births in his clinic resulted from the use of frozen sperm. Sherman's experience established the frozen-storage technique as a simple, efficient way of storing human sperm.

What are the planned applications for artificial insemination? Initially the purpose of freezing sperm was for the treatment of infertility. In 10 to 15 per cent of infertile couples the man is entirely responsible. One of the well-known causes of male sterility is mumps, a common harmless disease in children but capable of devastating destruction of testicular tissue in the adult male, often resulting in nearly complete sterility. Sperm from such men can be collected over a long period of time, frozen, concentrated, and injected artificially into the vagina, thus raising the chances of a successful pregnancy. By this method the parents remain the true parents;

only *their* genes contribute to the genetic makeup of the child.

With the popularization of vasectomy as a method of contraception, deep freezing of sperm provides a form of "fertility insurance." In most cases vasectomy is an irreversible surgical operation and creates legitimate concerns in many men about their future parental chances if an existing marriage ends in divorce or the death of the wife. Deep freezing of sperm provides a "hedge" against permanent sterility.

Increasing demand for sperm storage has resulted, not surprisingly, in the establishment of frozen-sperm banks. The first such bank, established in 1953 at the University of Iowa, is one of nine noncommercial sperm banks located in university hospitals or clinics across the nation. In 1970 the first commercial frozen-human-sperm bank opened in Saint Paul, Minnesota, followed by two others in San Francisco and New York.

What makes the whole issue of frozen-sperm banks of compelling interest is the general cloak of secrecy surrounding artificial insemination. Although no laws prohibit it in any way, AID registers do not exist in any country, nor are records compiled as to the recipients of the procedure or guidelines for its application. In addition, within the last three years the demand for artificial insemination has increased astronomically. With this increasing demand, all the storage banks have broadened their scope to the extent that very few other resources are now expended on the treatment of infertility within marriages, i.e., a husband's sperm used to fertilize his wife. Rather, a "sperm market" has come into existence, relying heavily on paid donors (the sperm used for insemination comes from someone paid anywhere from $10 to $50 per specimen). In the words of Mark Frankel, a research associate at the Program of Policy Studies in Science and Technology of the George Washington University, "At the present time practically anyone with sufficient funds, some liquid nitrogen, and the proper equipment can open a semen bank."

In 1971 Frankel began an investigation into frozen-semen banking in the United States. Published in December 1972 as *The Public Policy Dimensions of Artificial Insemination in Human Semen Cryobanking*, it is the first critical study ever done on sperm banks. Frankel started out by asking each frozen-sperm bank operating in the United States about its methods of selecting semen donors. To his surprise, Frankel discovered that no standard procedures existed. "While all the banks attempt to match the donor and recipient with respect to their physical characteristics, only about one-third report using some type of intelligence matching." Soon Frankel discovered other startling discrepancies: some banks took detailed medical and genetic histories of their donors, others did not; some required blood tests, others did not; some demanded screening tests and chromosome analysis for possible genetic abnormalities, others did not—in essence his data pointed to the "emergence of an industry without guidelines or a clearly perceived sense of direction." Even in the most fundamental matter of all—collection and storage—the banks have no standard policy. One used plastic ampoules, another glass ampoules, still another small plastic straws. Nor did any comparative research form the basis for the method of storage selected. Despite the obvious importance of establishing an optimum method of storage and standardization in the different clinics, the choice of methods still remained entirely up to the individual banks.

Some understanding of the implication of Frankel's findings can be gained by comparison with another donor-recipient relationship: blood. In England over 90 per cent of the blood is given free. In the United States 90 per cent of the blood has a price tag on it. Instead of raising the "quality" of the blood, the economical factor has wreaked havoc on our system of blood "donation." The Center for Disease Control in Atlanta estimates that some thirty-five hundred deaths per year are caused by hepatitis resulting from transfusions of infected blood. Statistics show that the rate of hepatitis in the blood of paid "donors" is ten times that of volunteers. This is not surprising, since the paid "donors" consist to a large extent of groups with a higher than average incidence of hepatitis. Included in these groups are alcoholics and drug addicts who "donate" blood again and again to support addiction or in many cases for just plain survival. As things now stand, there is no legislation preventing a similar development in the sperm market.

Almost incredible to contemplate is the naiveté of the average subscriber to sperm banks. Despite scientific demonstrations going back a hundred years or more that stress the importance of genes in determining physical and even mental characteristics, seemingly rational people are accepting on faith the idea that proper screening has been carried out on the genetic material that is going to be used to make their children. Although most would scruple at marrying a drug addict or a confirmed alcoholic, similar reservations appear nonexistent when it comes to creating a child with the genes of addicts or alcoholics.* Admittedly the relative contribution of genetics and environment to the development of addiction is still unsettled question. Despite these uncertainties, however, many are proceeding on the assumption that it is *all* environmental.

Nor is such a casual attitude restricted to the couples concerned. An obstetrician of international reputation recently told me he routinely "supplemented" a husband's sperm with donor material to bring the number of sperm to a high enough level to guarantee fertilization. "It's all right," he said, "because I know the sperm is gotten from donors who are graduate students." Such is the state of donor investigation in at least one university medical center!

One thing we can conclude from this is that our attitude toward the contribution of genetic inheritance to human destiny, always a curious one, is now, as with Alice's experience in Wonderland, getting "curiouser and curiouser." Today, for the most part, culture is given priority over heredity as the major influence on why people behave as they do, or on how long they will live, or what diseases they will contract over a lifetime. But that attitude may have to change in the light of new scientific evidence. Within the last ten years, several studies on biological relatives reared apart have proved that

---

* This is not to imply that drug addiction or alcoholism is entirely genetic. Nevertheless, most behavioral scientists, if they're frank about it, will admit that we're presently uncertain as to the exact contribution of genetic makeup to behavioral abnormalities. In the case of schizophrenia, appreciation of the genetic "loading" seems to be increasing (see page 72).

the genetic influence on behavior and social adaptability, for instance, is more powerful than previously imagined.

In a comprehensive investigation begun in 1959 and not completely finished even today, Dr. Seymour Kety, a professor of psychiatry at the Harvard Medical School, surveyed the incidence of schizophrenia among the genetic relatives of Danish children given up at birth for adoption. Using the detailed, encyclopedic *Medical Registry* kept in Copenhagen, Dr. Kety was able in most cases to trace these persons from their birth until the present (it must be remembered that throughout their lives they had no contact with their genetic relatives). Of the adopted children who became schizophrenic, more than half had schizophrenia somewhere in the genetic family, sometimes as close as a brother or sister, at other times as distant as a second cousin; the incidence of schizophrenia in their adopted families, however, was no higher than in the population at large. Genetic inheritance and not environment was thus prominent in the later development of schizophrenia in these cases.

Similar studies concerning people prone to or suffering from infectious diseases, heart disease, certain kinds of cancer, and hypertension all point to the importance of genetic inheritance. At the same time, the biomedical technology of AID is providing us with the means of blotting out the idea that one's parentage is a crucial determinant of one's physical and mental health.

We must remember that genetic inheritance has never been rigidly predictable. Even if we take the extreme position that all of us are *totally* conditioned by our genes, we are still faced with the fact that nobody has intentionally arranged the genes the way we find them. The genetic configuration of each one of us is "random" insofar as no one can possibly know *everything* about the genes of one's parents. This is a controlled randomness: a child's physical and mental characteristics are closer to those of his parents or other near relatives than they are to a stranger's. AID increases the randomness by drawing from an anonymous "gene pool," and by encouraging the idea that somehow it is so important for an infertile couple to have a child that they can forego consideration of their very biology.

Once again the message comes across that environment is more important than genetic inheritance, all at a time when basic genetic research is fashioning a counter-message: to a large extent, genes are destiny.

Most important, the genetic technology leading to AID is proceeding independently of any overall assessment of the long-term human consequences of these procedures. Once again, for some scientists at least, what can be done *must* be done. But the further development of AID as an embryo transfer need not be inevitable. For one thing, population studies cast serious doubts on the wisdom of funding any technology that results in an increase in the birthrate.

Despite the overwhelming importance of these issues for all of us, decisions regarding the funding and encouragement of further research along these lines has been so far discussed by "committees" composed entirely of scientists and research workers. For years, they alone have been deciding on questions regarding the further development of embryo-transfer techniques and AID banks. The questions have been discussed as "scientific ones," stripped of their important social consequences. I think it is obvious that, here, applied genetics is posing questions not capable of resolution within the scientific establishments. They are personal and social questions.

Stated at its simplest, "How much tampering do we want with processes of human sexuality and reproduction?" And, "How much power over our genes are we willing to relinquish to biotechnical specialists?"

The Third Wish

Sharon Berstein was eight months' pregnant before she ever thought of the possibility that something might be wrong with her baby. One reads about mongols, of course, but somehow that sort of thing only happens to other people.

A graduate student in economics, Sharon married late, at thirty-three, and postponed her first child until her Ph.D. dissertation was finished, by which time she was thirty-five. The pregnancy was relatively easy, some nausea early on, some "blue periods," but still everything going fairly smoothly. It was in a woman's magazine that Sharon first read of the increased incidence of mongols born to older mothers. "From that moment on, I worried almost constantly about my baby."

The birth of Terry turned out to be the confirmation of Sharon's worst fear. She didn't need to be told that Terry wasn't normal. The broad short head, the flat spadelike hands with short fingers, the slanting eyes—Sharon was able to anticipate the doctor's diagnosis. "He's a mongol, isn't he?"

Sharon Berstein is one of nearly twenty thousand women a year in the United States who give birth to children with a genetic disease of the chromosomes such as mongolism. The medical term for mongolism is Down's syndrome. Typically, it occurs in mothers like Sharon who are older than the average at the time of delivery. (Only about 2 per cent of infants are born to mothers over forty. These same mothers provide nearly 20 per cent of all mongols born in a given year.) If you include slightly younger mothers like Sharon, you find them accounting for a little over 10 per cent of all births but about 45 per cent of all the children with Down's syndrome. In other words, almost half the total number of mongoloids are born to mothers thirty-five years of age or over.

Down's syndrome involves an abnormality in the number or structure of the chromosomes. Normally the chromosomes are paired, twenty-three contributed from each parent, resulting in forty-six chromosomes capable of identification by special staining techniques. Along the length of the chromosomes are the genes, the blueprints for the synthesis of millions of enzymes responsible for growth. While these genes usually remain confined to one or the other chromosome and in fact can be mapped according to location, in genetic disorders like Down's syndrome a segment of chromosome number twenty-one becomes detached and hooked on to chromosome number fifteen. This is a fifteen–twenty-one translocation, one cause of mongolism. Another cause is the duplication of chromosome number twenty-one in either the husband's sperm cell or the wife's egg, resulting in three chromosomes at the twenty-one position instead of only two: trisomy.

Diagnosis of Down's syndrome depends on obtaining sample cells of the fetus and staining them with a special stain. The method for doing this, developed only in the last twenty years, is an illustration of the promise and peril of applied genetics. While doubts may exist regarding the diagnosis before birth of other genetic disorders, Down's syndrome provides the model for an efficient, almost 100 per cent accurate, diagnosis of the genetic disease in the womb. It all involves examination of fluid in the uterus surrounding the fetus. This is known as amniotic fluid, and the method for its collection is amniocentesis.

Let me say just a little about amniocentesis, or I'm afraid much of what I'll say later won't make much sense. During its growth in the uterus, the fetus remains surrounded by a fluid-filled amniotic sac. Occasionally, in diseased states, the amniotic fluid contained in the sac can accumulate to dangerous proportions, requiring its withdrawal via a puncture of the amniotic sac. Originally performed over a century ago, this procedure still constitutes a reasonable treatment for excessive amniotic fluid: polyhydramnios.

About twenty years ago, a British investigator carried out the first sampling of amniotic fluid for the purpose of finding out something about the condition of the fetus. Since the fetus is completely contained within the amniotic sac, he reasoned that the cells of the fluid must be of fetal origin and could be used to foretell some of the fetal characteristics. All further refinements in the technique of amniocentesis are based on this reasoning.

The actual data obtainable from amniocentesis, however, have accumulated very slowly, almost all of them within the last eight years. It wasn't until 1966 that amniotic fluid was first used to grow cells for chromosome studies. Two years later came the first demonstration of genetically determined deficiencies in enzymes, specialized protein chemicals that trigger key body reactions leading to normal growth and development. Each succeeding year has seen more and more sophisticated biochemical analysis of the components of amniotic fluid.

To get the amniotic fluid for analysis requires the insertion of a needle into the womb at about sixteen weeks of pregnancy. The amniotic fluid is withdrawn through the needle and examined in the laboratory. From chromosome analysis such diseases as Down's syndrome can then be diagnosed; also, the sex of the fetus can be determined and is of extreme importance in those diseases that are sex linked, that occur only in males or only in females. With increasing knowledge of the biochemistry of certain genetic disorders, we have discovered that most genetic diseases are not chromosomal in character at all, but are caused by deficiencies in one or more enzymes. Today, hundreds of genetic diseases, which result in varying degrees of physical and mental defects, are known. And there is no reason to doubt that the list will continue to grow of genetic diseases potentially diagnosable prior to birth by amniocentesis.

The performance of an amniocentesis is relatively simple. From the beginning, however, certain problems have limited its usefulness. First, there is a small but definite risk (between 1 and 5 per cent, depending on the surgeon) either that the procedure will injure the fetus directly by an ill-placed needle insertion or that a spontaneous abortion will be stimulated. Second, the information provided by amniocentesis is only as precise as the questions asked. In other words, a laboratory capable of analyzing chromosomes and twenty-eight enzymes is much better than one equipped to analyze chromosomes and only fifteen or twenty enzymes. So far, these analyses are available only at the large hospitals and other major medical centers. Third, the usefulness of amniocentesis is complicated somewhat by the resulting lapse of time needed before the fetal cells can grow in tissue culture. This can range from seven to twelve weeks which, when added to the optimal period for the performance of amniocentesis, can reach twenty-three to twenty-eight weeks after the start of pregnancy, long past the allowable time for elective abortion if it is wanted or needed. Finally, there is the question of the accuracy of the information obtained from amniotic fluid. In the case of Down's syndrome the accuracy is virtually 100 per cent, but with other chromosome abnormalities the predictability is not that good. And perfectly normal individuals have been found to possess chromosome abnormalities that usually result in genetic defects.

Despite these problems, the use of amniocentesis in the diagnosis of Down's syndrome represents applied genetics at its best. The difficulties arise in deciding what use should be made of the knowledge that the technique supplies—for example, that a yet unborn child has Down's syndrome with its accompanying 95 per cent chance of severe retardation and 5 per cent chance of mild to moderate degrees of retardation.

The most obvious course is abortion. Some feel that, theoretically at least, Down's syndrome could be abolished if all pregnancies of risk were monitored by amniotic-fluid examination and all fetuses discovered to have Down's syndrome were aborted.

One doctor who holds to this view is Cecil B. Jacobson, chief of the Reproductive Genetics Unit at the George Washington University Hospital in Washington, D.C., and one of the early developers of amniocentesis as a tool of the new genetics. He told me he had completed more than seven hundred amniocenteses, the largest number by any single person in the world. "You show me just one mongoloid that has an educable IQ," he exclaimed, as we discussed the risks and dangers of mongolism. "I've never seen even one in my experience with over eight hundred mongols in the District of Columbia. I've known people to be so frightened by mongolism that they won't undergo pregnancy without amniocentesis. I feel I should provide them with this procedure if they ask for it. The only alternative is to tell them not to have children at all. Believe me, the consequences of telling people not to have children are dire."

Jacobson has been caught in a cross fire in the last few years, in part because of his controversial experiments in artificial fertilization. But equally contributory to the notoriety is a blustering tendency to make blunt, verbal attacks on the arguments of those who haven't done what he considers their intellectual homework.

"The mongol question is just the most superficial part of the whole problem. I can't imagine any reasonably responsible person arguing against the abortion of mongols. But I'd like to take the thing a few steps further. Would you, for instance, want to conceive a child who will die of cancer at age forty if the tendency for the development of cancer can be shown before birth? Naturally, at this point we're not able to do that. But if we could tell what fetuses are going to be afflicted with cancer in their forties or fifties, I would be for aborting them now. That would eliminate some types of cancer forever."

Dr. Jacobson is outrageous, and he knows it. He is also deeply committed, and impatient with what he calls the misplaced sentimentalism of many of his colleagues. To him, many of the bioethical questions are "pseudo questions," delaying what he considers to be inevitable. His impatience stems from a sincere desire to get on with the business of screening the members of a very special and important club: the next one or two generations. "The final arbiter of what children should be born are the parents themselves," he said. "Only they know what is best for their marriage. Take the issue of sex determination, for instance. I don't have any hesitation in cooperating with an abortion if both parents want only girls and the current pregnancy tests out by amniocentesis to be a boy. I just don't recognize any absolutes here."

In essence Dr. Jacobson and an increasing number of other experts in this field see parents as consumers, alternately selecting and rejecting various possible variations in children. Those who wish only blue-eyed children, for instance, might someday be provided with the technology needed to bring this about. "The Supreme Court decision on abortion has come down squarely on the side of whatever desires the woman, or the couple, have about what kind of children they're going to produce. The real question now is whether people are going to be willing to come to grips with some of the really tough questions."

One of the tough questions Dr. Jacobson referred to is

what to do about the alarming number of carriers of genetic diseases that are brought to light through the use of techniques like amniocentesis. As of this moment amniocentesis is used primarily for the detection of fetuses (known as homozygotes) with the fully expressed forms of genetic disease. Other fetuses from the same parents may have narrowly missed that same genetic fate by a lucky combination of healthy genes that have suppressed or eliminated the harmful ones. Years later, however, those children may pass on the harmful genes to *their* children, who may not be so lucky. Such people are "carriers"; if they happen to marry another carrier, there is at least a one-in-four risk of producing children with the fully developed disease. The most frightening thing about the "carrier state" is its silence. Any one of us may be a biological time bomb capable of living a normal life but passing on to our children a lethal or crippling genetic disease.

It is conservatively estimated that each person carries anywhere from four to eight defective genes which, when combined with a mate possessing those same unfavorable genes, can result in genetic disease. Such combinations are rare simply because everybody has different types of "bad genes" whose expression is prevented by the presence of a dominant healthy gene. Such a person's genetic "formula" is $Nn: N$ is a dominant gene and n a recessive abnormal one whose expression is blocked by the N or normal gene. If two such Nn people marry, there is a one-in-four chance that their children will be $nn:$ the fully expressed genetic disease that can result in death or disability. People with two completely normal genes (NN) are called homozygotes; those with Nn are called heterozygotes.

Obviously, as the number of heterozygotes increase, the chances of producing nn individuals increases accordingly. These heterozygotes are popularly known by geneticists as "silent carriers": they're not abnormal themselves but carry a recessive gene that can result in abnormality, given a mate with a similar Nn genetic makeup. The tough question is what to do about the carriers. Dr. Jacobson has an answer to this dilemma: "Take a woman in a family of hemophiliacs. She doesn't have hemophilia because women don't get it. They pass it on to their sons. Hemophilia is sex-linked. The daughters of this woman will be just like Mom: a carrier for hemophilia passing the fully developed hemophilia to fifty per cent of their sons. Now we're just at the point that people are beginning to accept the fact that all of the male fetuses of such a woman should be aborted. Even though only half of them will have hemophilia, there is no way at this time of telling which ones, so why take a chance? I think we're eventually going to come to the point where we'll abort more and more of the females as well. Unfortunately, only by aborting normal people in this generation can we spare the next generation from the burden of some forms of genetic disease."

Dr. Jacobson points out that females born to a "carrier" for hemophilia should themselves undergo amniocentesis for every pregnancy and an untold number of abortions of male fetuses. "Believe me, this kind of mental anguish has a disastrous effect on people's marriages and mental health. I've been noting that among women who have had repeated episodes of amniocentesis followed by abortion for genetic disease there is a growing unwillingness to pass on this misery to their female children."

What will the future hold for genetic carriers? At this point nobody knows. But Dr. Jacobson has obviously thought very carefully about the general direction he thinks applied genetics should be taking. "If you ask a hundred couples each to give you three wishes for their children," he says, "you get a lot of different answers. I'm certain in the near future everybody's third wish is going to be, 'I wish my child to be able to some day give birth to totally normal children.' I want to help bring that wish to a fulfillment."

How close are we to bringing Cecil Jacobson's third wish about? To find out, I visited Guy's Hospital in London and spoke with Dr. Jack Singer, senior lecturer in human genetics and physician to the Genetic Screening Unit. He explained how the genetics unit at Guy's works: "First, as many spontaneous abortions as possible are studied for abnormalities in the chromosomes. That means as soon as a woman in London loses a baby we set about trying to find out if a chromosome abnormality might have caused the abortion. The mother is contacted and questioned about infections, exposure to X rays, and accidents—all known to increase the incidence of abnormal chromosomes. Once these factors are eliminated we are left with a large group of women for whom a cause can't be found for their abnormal chromosomes. It is this group we focus attention on."

Dr. Singer went on to explain the scope of the Genetic Screening Unit's activities: "Some abnormal chromosomes are spread throughout the entire family, extending to aunts, uncles, and cousins. Most of these people are normal but they should be studied to see if they run a higher risk of producing a deformed child. Take, for example, the fifteen–twenty-one translocation. If we discover a woman with this translocated chromosome we check her parents, brothers, sisters, aunts, uncles . . . in all about fifty people sometimes have to be contacted. Blood specimens are taken from all of them and examined for evidence of the fifteen–twenty-one abnormality. Those found to have it, although normal themselves, have a higher than average risk of about twenty-five per cent versus four-tenths of one per cent, approximately a hundredfold increase, of producing a defective child. The pregnancies from these people should have amniocentesis."

Within the last five years, two major advances in prenatal diagnosis have been achieved. It is now possible after amniocentesis to separate the mother's cells from the fetal cells with increasing precision, thus refining the ability to detect a defective child. From the first application of the amniocentesis technique, many scientists have been worried about mistaking the fetal cells for some of the mother's own cells, which are also found in the amniotic fluid. But with further refinements in the technique of identifying cell types, the accuracy of diagnosis is now approaching 100 per cent. (One gynecologist, however, painfully recalls receiving in the mail the foreskin of an infant he had predicted by amniocentesis to be a girl.)

The second major advance involves the detection of a chemical, Alpha feto protein, which leaks out of the damaged fetal nervous system and passes into the mother's bloodstream, where it can be detected and measured. This is the first screening test developed that uses blood rather than amniotic fluid. It is easy, dependable, and eliminates the 1 to 5 per cent complication risk of amniocentesis.

But laboratory tests are only half the work of genetic clinics. In addition, formal genetic counseling is offered. Genetic counseling, simply stated, is the application of genetic knowledge to individual pregnancies in order to predict defective offspring. The greatest number of people coming for genetic counseling are parents of one or more defective children. "Will it happen again?" is the question they want answered, and it is an anguishing question. "Initially the earliest genetic counselors were a bit like bookmakers," says Dr. Singer. "The counselor sat down with the parents, took a careful family history on both sides, and drew up a family tree—a pedigree going back as far as possible. He was then able to compute the odds of a defect's being hereditary, first of all, and secondly, of its occurring again. But in the last ten or fifteen years the scope of applied genetics has changed drastically. We now have specialized tests to detect ahead of time a large number of genetic diseases. We're much more concerned now than previously with determining the causes of these abnormalities and with developing treatments where possible. Treatment, unfortunately, isn't available except for a small number of genetic diseases, and the emphasis must remain on prevention by prenatal diagnosis and abortion."

Prevention of genetic disease is a shared goal of counselor and clients alike. Yet the practical application of this goal seems fraught with difficulties. "The real problem involves the change in the counselor's role," states Dr. Singer. "Is he an information-giver, as he was in the past? Should he say, 'The tests indicate there is the likelihood of a defective child: make up your own mind'? Or should he intrude his own values and say, 'The risk is too high and I'd advise you to have an abortion'? The genetic counselor shouldn't put himself in the role of God, and yet many times this is what the parents want: someone to tell them what they should do."

One thing fostering such dependence may be the ever increasing knowledge gap between counselor and client. Applied genetics, even at its simplest, is not readily grasped by the nonspecialist. In a study done at St. Christopher's Hospital in Philadelphia, only 19 per cent of the parents counseled regarding a genetic disease were able to express in writing a basic understanding of it—this after months of indoctrination by individual counselors, group discussions, and the reading of pamphlets written in laymen's language. "The issues involved are just too emotionally charged for the parents to take anything like an objective attitude," continues Dr. Singer. "Distortions and misunderstandings are inevitable."

The genetic counselors at Guy's are physicians who have been specially trained in the science of human genetics. The qualifications and training of similar specialists elsewhere in the world vary immensely: there are genetic superspecialists like Dr. Singer, a former Rockefeller Foundation scholar, and there are the graduates of a small girl's college in the United States that offers a master's degree in genetic counseling. At the present time there are no boards or specialized credentials in the United States or England prerequisite to anyone offering services as a "genetic counselor." "A genetic unit capable of testing and counseling parents is a responsibility not to be taken lightly," says Dr. Singer. "In fact, if a full complement of specialists employed full time under the direction of a fully trained geneticist is not available, a hospital or clinic is better off not offering any services at all. The risk of mistakes in diagnosis is just too serious."

Two examples of difficulty in diagnosis are provided by "blighted ova" and "balanced carriers." "Consider a twin pregnancy, with one of the fetuses normal, the other a mongol," Dr. Singer explains. "Both are developing up to a certain point, when the mongol fetus dies, leaving only the perfectly normal fetus. A few cells from the dead mongol fetus, known as a blighted ovum, may be obtained by amniocentesis. These abnormal cells may cause the counselor to misdiagnose the normal baby as a mongol and lead to the termination of a normal pregnancy. Admittedly this is rare, but rare things happen, and almost any genetic unit, if they're frank about it, will tell you of such unfortunate experiences.

"The balanced-carrier situation points up the difficulty involved in something like amniocentesis where you don't have a patient you can see and you have to make a judgment on incomplete evidence because you aren't dealing directly with the patient. Sometimes when the chromosomes of the parents are examined, an abnormality is found which might indicate mental retardation, for instance. To test that out all you have to do is look at the parents, talk to them, do psychological testing if necessary, and you have your answer. They're either retarded or they're not. If you get the same chromosome abnormality from an amniotic fluid sample, you can't test and examine the patient. Recently a perfectly normal woman was discovered to have a balanced chromosome that often is seen with the severely mentally retarded. Now if we do an amniocentesis on her next pregnancy and find the same chromosomal 'abnormality,' what do we do? The child may turn out to be just as normal as the mother. It might equally turn out to be retarded. There's simply no way at this point of making that distinction."

The demands on genetic units are rising at an astronomical rate. Referrals from family physicians, obstetricians, and social workers multiply as the list of genetically diagnosable diseases grows longer. The referrals for one genetic disease increased 50 per cent at Guy's Hospital over a six-month period in early 1973. Such increases are forcing immediate decision on priorities: what available resources should be invested in genetic units and for what purpose?

But this emphasis on the financial and manpower aspects bypasses what is probably the most fundamental question: when you get right down to it, how much does anybody really want to know about their genes? Dr. Robert Murray of Howard University in Washington, D.C., thinks they might want to know far less than some genetic counselors insist on telling them. "If I do not happen to know that my wife and I are carriers of a particular trait, we are free to go ahead and conceive our own natural children. We might be among the lucky ones and have our first two or three children . . . normal. On the other hand if we learned that we are carriers, our freedom to act would be compromised if we were concerned citizens. In this particular instance we would have greater freedom through ignorance."

As a further complication, genetic disease often affects many people in a family, some of whose members may share Dr. Murray's reluctance to be told any genetic "bad news." Take for instance, tylosis, a rare skin disease easily diagnosed by a mild rash found on the palms of the hands. What gives tylosis its grim importance is that people who suffer from it have a 75 per cent chance of eventually developing cancer of the esophagus. The skin lesions of tylosis are, in fact, "genetic markers" for the nearly always fatal cancer of the esophagus. Oh, yes, one more thing—tylosis runs in families.

What should the genetic counselor tell the relatives of a patient with tylosis? It seems obvious that the patient himself should be told of the necessity of preventive measures against the cancer. He should also be told of the corresponding risk for other family members, but beyond that, how far can the counselor go? What about telling other family members who haven't asked for advice as patients or clients?

These questions are not easy. They also touch on the relationship of a patient to his doctor (or, by extension, of a client to his counselor). Traditionally this relationship has been rigidly defined. The patient, desiring help with some physical or mental problem, goes to a specialist trained in the diagnosis and treatment of disease. Except in rare emergencies the doctor does not initiate the contact. (The ancient practice of quarantine, of course, rests on the assumption that the doctor has a right and duty under special circumstances to prevent the progress of disease to healthy people.) New and troubling are cases similar to tylosis where doctors must act on the basis of special knowledge to enlist unknowing and perhaps unwilling people into the role of "patients." And tylosis is one of the easy cases. After all, everybody concerned benefits from an early forewarning of impending cancer. With other examples, however, the benefits aren't so obvious.

If you ever met someone with testicular feminization, you probably never knew there was anything different about them. To all outward appearances they are perfectly normal women. Therein lies the problem. They're not women at all, but men; their chromosomes are clearly male, and in place of a uterus such people have a rudimentary sexual organ similar to the testes. Reproduction or menstruation is, of course, impossible. Most of them live out their lives without coming to medical attention simply because childless couples even today don't always find their way into a gynecologist's office. The usual reason for seeking help, however, is failure of the "woman" with testicular feminization to become pregnant after marriage. And they come to the doctor with all the anxieties and self-doubts that childlessness engenders.

The diagnosis of testicular feminization can be counted on to set off an emotional powder keg. What is at stake is no less than the patient's sexual identity. In a sense, she is not a *she* at all, but a *he*. No amount of tact can be guaranteed to save either the patient's marriage or sanity. And, as with tylosis, the patient with testicular feminization has a greatly increased chance of contacting a cancer, in this case cancer of those incomplete sexual organs. Accepted practice as well as common humanity demands the patient be informed, and the potentially cancerous organs be removed. But informed of what? That "she" is actually a "he"? Naturally, if a doctor is recommending major surgery he has to come up with a reasonable explanation of what is wrong. Some doctors have avoided the issue in the past by reliance on ambiguity and medical mumbo jumbo to reassure the individual patient.

To complicate things further, however, the patient's relatives are also at risk for the same problem. Perhaps the patient has two sisters aged ten and fourteen. There is a very real chance that one or even both of these normally appearing females are in fact further instances of people with testicular feminization. Suddenly the whole thing is not simply the private matter of one patient. We are talking about the rights of her two sisters to be spared the future development of a potentially preventable cancer. We are talking of the rights of two as yet unknown husbands to marry genetically normal women capable of producing children. In short, we are talking of the rights of numerous people to be informed so that they can make intelligent decisions; at the same time we are talking about information that can act like napalm on marriages, family solidarity, and sexual identity.

What Price
the Perfect Baby?

In 1972 a divinity student in a major American seminary decided against taking his newly born mongol son home from the hospital. In addition to mongolism, the infant suffered from a duodenal atresia: an easily corrected constriction of the outlet from the stomach. The student and his wife, after deciding against surgery, visited the infant daily to take photographs up until the child's death at seventeen days. "I wouldn't take anything in the world for the opportunity I've had to make this decision," said the student. "I know we've made the right decision."

■ In Washington, D.C., the mother of a mentally retarded son visited a genetic counseling unit for amniocentesis when she became pregnant again, for she and her husband were anxious to prevent the birth of another genetically abnormal child. Upon returning home she found her retarded son hiding in a closet. Over the next few days he had trouble sleeping because of nightmares that someone was trying to hurt him.

These are only two results of the recent change in our attitudes toward the genetically defective. What are the long-term implications of applied genetics? In our search for the perfect baby, just what price are we prepared to pay?

I discussed this with Dr. John Fletcher, co-chairman of the Institute of Society, Ethics, and the Life Sciences, Study Group on Genetic Screening and Counseling. A man who speaks in a charming Southern accent that manages to combine gentleness with exquisite politeness, Dr. Fletcher can instantly display the incisiveness of a master tactician when discussing the future of applied genetics. While others have speculated about where genetic technology may be taking us, Dr. Fletcher is one of the few who has done something about finding out the answers. "In the past, doctors and society in general were geared toward helping parents to accept a defective child as a substitute for the healthy one they had hoped for," he remarked to me. "This was possible because of religious and moral factors but also because nothing could be done about the genetically defective anyway. I was interested in studying the effect made by applied genetics on the family unit, particularly the bond between parent and child."

Dr. Fletcher studied twenty-five couples of widely differing social and ethnic backgrounds. All the couples had come for genetic counseling when the wife asked for amniocentesis with the intention of aborting any fetus discovered to be abnormal. More than half the couples came to the counseling unit because they had previously borne defective children. The next largest group consisted of older couples anxious to avoid the risk of a mongoloid child. "This is the first generation of parents in history who are already crossing a borderline of decision making, venturing out to use the knowledge obtainable from prenatal diagnosis of genetic disease in their newborn children." Thus the first stage of genetic medicine is already being institutionalized as amniocentesis is being used more routinely. "If one thing could be said to characterize these highly diverse people, it was a strong motivation to have children and to go to extraordinary lengths to exercise responsible parenthood," continued Dr. Fletcher. But this strong desire for a healthy child combined with a willingness to abort genetically defective children resulted, he thought, in "moral suffering" of the highest order. "There is often an unusual sense of shame and guilt associated with genetic disease which I have come to call 'cosmic guilt.' We can't underestimate this in dealing with those people who know there's something the matter with their genes." One father told him, "We have an obligation to our children before they are born; you can't turn your back on the future." Another father said, "I couldn't go through it again. . . . It is not doing anything for the child, or for society, to be born so sickly." After the results of amniocentesis were reported, all those told of genetic abnormality opted for abortion. In addition, all the volunteers then underwent sterilization.

The reasons given for the drastic step of sterilization were highly personal and related to the feelings of emotional strain. "I just can't go through this again," one mother told Dr. Fletcher. In the words of another mother, "You spend all your life looking at the pictures of pretty babies and their mothers and growing up thinking that will be you. It is pretty gruesome when you're the one who is different."

So far, Dr. Fletcher's findings seemed neither unusual nor unexpected, given the anguishing nature of the problems. What *was* unusual was the subtle transformation he observed in the relationships of the parents with their own children, both normal and genetically defective. As one parent put it, "One day it hit me: What is Johnny going to think about us now? Is he going to wonder, 'What would Mommy and Daddy have done if something had been wrong with *me*?'" Similar feelings were reported by the other parents. Dr. Fletcher found evidence that the trusting relationship of the couples toward their living children was permanently altered by the experience of genetic counseling and amniocentesis. "Even if the diagnosis given by genetic investigation were negative," Dr. Fletcher said, "you have nonetheless entertained the idea of the death of your baby. To contemplate the death of your baby in the third month of pregnancy changes very seriously the attitude we, as a society, usually have toward our babies."

Dr. Fletcher bases his few tentative conclusions both on the results of his small study and on Erik Erikson's concept of the "basic trust" that must exist between parent and child. Still, he acknowledges that the tendency to reject the unfit is nothing new. In fact, he says, "The tendency of parents and doctors to reject the genetically defective is an all too natural one. It's only after hundreds of years that we've been able to establish social attitudes toward the care of defective persons. I don't want to see amniocentesis and applied genetics destroying our capacity for support and compassion for those who don't measure up to our norms."

Dr. Fletcher's findings have a profound implication regarding our future attitudes toward illness in general. If an infant born with a cleft palate is unthinkable for some parents, what will the attitude of those same parents be to another child who develops leukemia at the age of five? What will be our attitudes in the next decade toward the sick? the permanently disabled? the incurable? How will we respond to those who are now alive with genetic defects but who could have been aborted? Are we on the threshold of an era when "second-class citizens" and "nonpersons" will be distinguished from the rest of us? For Dr. Leon Kass, the prospect is a real and frightening one. "A child with genetic defect, born at a time when most of his potential fellow sufferers were destroyed prenatally, is liable to be looked upon by the community as one unfit to be alive, as a second-class (or even lower) human type. He may seem a person who need not have been, and who would not have been if only someone had gotten to him in time."

Dr. Kass's manner is ordered, low key, and refreshingly free of cant. Yet his visions of what might come on the genetic horizon scared the hell out of me when I confronted (for the first time) the logical extension of the new genetics. "It must always be remembered that we shall always have abnormals—some who escape detection or whose disease is undetectable *in utero*," he told me. (Other groups include those with new mutations of the genes, birth injuries, accidents, maltreatment, or disease.) All of them, according to Dr. Kass, will require care and protection. "The existence of defectives cannot be prevented. Is it not likely that our principle with respect to these people will change from 'we try harder' to 'why accept second best'?"

Dr. Kass fears that the idea of the "unwanted because abnormal child" may become a self-fulfilling prophecy whose consequences are worse than the abnormality itself. "In fact, it is the natural standard which may be the most dangerous one, in that it leads most directly to the idea that there are second-class human beings and subhuman beings. 'Defectives should not be born' is a principle without limit."

Warning: Genetics May Be Hazardous to Your Health

Within the next decade genetic technology can be expected to affect our daily lives in the most intimate ways imaginable. Before us is the prospect of such things as mass screening a whole generation for hundreds, perhaps even thousands, of genetic disorders. Indeed the possibilities are mind boggling. But overemphasis on the scientific obscures the question of the social applications and consequences of the new genetic technologies. Consider for a moment a few applications of genetics within our recent past:

In 1965 Dr. Patricia Jacobs reported an association between violent behavior and the chromosome sex abnormality XYY. Studying inmates of Carstairs Maximum Security Hospital in Scotland, she detected an extra Y chromosome in 3.6 per cent of the inmates confined for violent and severely "socially deviant behavior." When she compared the figures to a "normal" group, she detected only 5 XYYs in 3500 consecutive male infants (0.14 per cent) and *no* XYYs in 2040 "normal" adult males. On the basis of these findings, Dr. Jacobs generated a hypothesis linking an extra Y chromosome and a tendency to "criminality."

Widespread publicity was given the Carstairs work when Richard Speck, the Chicago mass murderer of nine nurses, was reported by chromosome analysis to be an XYY. The tattoo Speck had on his arm, "Born to Raise Hell," supported an emerging popular stereotype that XYY individuals were physically aggressive and violent. It was suggested in some circles that mass screening of infants at birth for the detection of XYYs could identify future criminals and the "socially deviant."

In 1970 technology provided a means of applying Dr. Jacobs' hypothesis to large groups of people. Researchers on leukemia at Harvard and at the Karolinska Institute in Stockholm developed special fluorescent stains which preferentially dyed the Y or male chromosome, making it possible to read chromosome patterns from cells such as those from the buccal mucosa, the inner lining of the cheek. This new technique provided a rapid screening of newborns as well as adults with a history of criminality or impulse-control problems. All was in readiness for the detection of possible crimes ten, twenty, maybe even thirty years before their commission. If the potential criminal could be spotted early enough, it was reasoned, who could say how much future violence could be averted?

Only one thing prevented the setting up of vast screening programs for XYY males: follow-up studies by other investigators did not support Dr. Jacobs' conclusions. Studies in prisons and mental hospitals in England, the United States, Denmark, and France concluded that XYYs did not appear to be concentrated among the most dangerous, violent, or physically aggressive inmates. The offenses committed by them were in general similar to or less serious than those committed by normal XY males. In addition, a larger number of XYYs were found in the general population than had been reported by Dr. Jacobs' study. Businessmen, clergymen, automobile assembly-line workers—in such groups as these XYY males began showing up, and none of them had any history of "violent" or "socially deviant" behavior. In a comprehensive study, "Behavioral Implications of the Human XYY Genotype," published in *Science* in January 1973, Dr. Ernest Hook concluded that the XYY-criminality association had not been proved, but must wait until "a large prospectively ascertained group is studied with suitable precautions."

What is clear from this history is that a movement in favor of worldwide screening for a phony genetic "disease" was only narrowly avoided. For a short period in the late 1960s an atypical chromosome pattern (whose significance is still to be assessed) was flaunted as an indicator of criminality. There are precedents for such premature and incorrect genetic conclusions. And a similar experience has occurred within the last three years concerning sickle-cell trait.

If you ask the average black man what sickle-cell trait is, he'll more than likely tell you something like this: "Sickle-cell trait is a mild form of the disease sickle-cell anemia. Both are found mostly in blacks. The trait is not as bad as the sickle-cell anemia; you don't die early; you can do most of the things other people can do; but still you've got a mild form of sickle-cell anemia." The implication is that people with sickle-cell trait suffer from a "genetic disease" transmitted from one generation to another among blacks.

A typical advertisement for the purpose of raising money for sickle-cell research described the sickle-cell disease: "It's a killer. One out of every ten Black Americans carries a blood trait that threatens to cripple or kill. It's called Sickle Cell Disease because it creates deformed 'sickle shaped' red blood cells. It can weaken those it doesn't kill. Even those with the milder form of Sickle Cell Disease—the trait—suffer. Usually they must avoid strenuous activities and consult the doctor on a regular basis." Certainly the reader of this rather grim advertisement would be led to consider sickle-cell trait as a "disease," a genetic curse which, though somewhat milder than sickle-cell anemia, might do him in if appropriate precautions weren't taken. Nothing could be further from the truth.

"Such an advertisement is outright irresponsible, because the facts are that the vast majority of sickle-cell-trait carriers are quite healthy: they are not weakened; and they do not need to see a physician regularly," according to Dr. Arno Motulsky of the Division of Medical Genetics at the University of Washington in Seattle. "Some inherited characteristics do not necessarily lead to disease. . . . The sickle-cell trait is a perfectly innocuous trait except under very unusual circumstances. Someone who has the trait is not sick; he or she is well. It is possible that screening programs may be doing more harm than good by implying ill health when it does not exist."

Dr. Motulsky backs up his contention with autopsy studies showing no difference among normals and sickle-cell-trait carriers and suggesting no difference in mortality from the "trait." Others go still further: Herman Lehman, professor of clinical biochemistry at Cambridge University, has said, "On the whole and for practical purposes one can assume that the sickle-cell trait is harmless."

Why is there this difference between orthodox scientific opinion and the more fatalistic view sold to the public in newspapers, magazines, and on television? To answer this, one must know a little bit about sickle-cell disease and a whole lot more about genetic myths.

The story of sickle-cell disease began in 1910 when J. B. Herrick, a hematologist, examined the blood of a seriously ill West Indian black student living in Chicago. Herrick described "peculiar elongated and sickle-shaped" red blood cells. It was soon found that the red blood cells of certain blacks, although perfectly normal under ordinary conditions, tended to assume a "sickle shape" when oxygen was reduced. This was first shown experimentally by removing red blood cells from these patients and subjecting the cells to reduced-oxygen conditions. By 1933 Dr. Lemuel W. Diggs and his associates distinguished between those patients in whom "sickling" of the red blood cell was associated with a profound disease (sickle-cell anemia) and others in whom the abnormality was a "harmless trait."

Almost all the manifestations of sickle-cell disease result from the clogging effect that the sickle-shaped red blood cells have within the blood vessels of the body. It's as if a smoothly flowing liquid were suddenly changed, developing the thickness of molasses or heavy-duty machine oil. The abnormal red cells clog the blood vessels leading to important organs such as the heart, brain, kidneys, and lungs. Deprived of their oxygen supply, these organs undergo cellular death, a process known as infarction. Sickle-cell "crisis" is the medical term for this death of cells and tissues in the body. The sickle cells can cause acute blockage of blood to the stomach, pneumonia, even heart attacks; it is also one of the most painful experiences imaginable. (Sometimes, pathetic and painless devastations can occur. One of my own patients, five years old, became blind when the blood vessels to the vital centers of the brain necessary for vision became blocked.)

That the sickling phenomenon was inherited was demonstrated as early as 1923. The presence of the full-fledged disease, sickle-cell anemia, required that both parents had the sickle-cell trait. In other words, the parents would be perfectly normal but their children victims of the dreaded anemia. Abnormal sickle cells are always present to some degree in those who suffer from sickle-cell anemia. If the oxygen level is lowered around them—such as occurs in high altitudes, in airplanes, or while scuba diving—60 to 80 per cent of the circulating blood cells may suddenly sickle and a crisis result. The person with sickle-cell trait, on the other hand, has no sickle cells present in the circulating blood. Only under conditions of extreme oxygen lack, and I emphasize the word *extreme,* do sickle cells begin to appear. African athletes with sickle-cell trait who underwent extremes of physical stress at high altitudes in the Mexican Olympic Games in 1968 did not experience any sickle-cell crises, and there have been no documented reports of a "crisis" developing during air flight in persons with sickle-cell trait.

But the strictly medical aspects do not even come close to being the full story of sickle-cell disease, which even into the mid-1960s was of interest to only a few dedicated researchers laboring in obscurity to find a cure for a little-known disease. It was with the achievement of some of the goals of the civil rights movement that sickle-cell disease suddenly became important. "We want to know how much money has been set aside for research into sickle-cell anemia and who controls the money," demanded the black clergyman and television personality David Eaton. Suddenly sickle-cell disease had become more than a disease. It was a testing ground to discover how much American society was really committed to civil rights. What could be a truer test of commitment to social equality than to donate funds for research on sickle-cell disease?

Overnight the black community's concern with sickle-cell disease turned into a preoccupation, almost an obsession, as a demand sprang up for more and more information about it. Who had it? What did it mean? "Sickle-cell disease is becoming a household word, albeit for the wrong reasons," wrote University of Colorado geneticist and pediatrician Herbert Lubs. By the early 1970s the amount of misinformation about sickle-cell disease reached almost epidemic proportions. Even such unlikely sources as the Black Panther newspaper carried a series of articles on sickle-cell anemia and what could be done about it. In the confusion and hustle, key distinctions between sickle-cell anemia and sickle-cell trait became blurred. Even among the well informed, knowledge of being a sickle-cell-trait carrier often proved disastrous. For instance, a Washington, D.C., television program on the sickle-cell issue emphasized the importance of each and every viewer having himself tested for the presence of the trait. To underscore the importance of this message, one enthusiastic and well-intentioned volunteer had her hemoglobin tested during the show. Thousands of viewers were party to her speechless amazement when she was told the test was positive. The implications for the wide dissemination of erroneous information can be roughly calculated from the fact that Washington is 70 per cent black. Who knows how many black viewers were persuaded by that show that sickle-cell trait was as dangerous as "cancer" or "stroke"?

Since 1970 at least twenty-nine states and the District of Columbia have enacted screening programs for sickle-cell anemia. The first laws, such as the one in Massachusetts, were passed "in a euphoria of enthusiasm," as Dr. Derek Robinson, deputy commissioner of the Department of Health, put it. Rather than asking for voluntary procedures, the need for compulsory measures was underscored. As a Washington city councilman, Harry S. Robinson, argued: "This is a trait and a disease that has been ignored. There is no cure but a family knowing the facts knows what steps to take. . . . I don't think we can get at the problem on a voluntary basis. There is too much apathy."

Already, most states have enacted subsequent legislation to repeal the hastily drawn-up compulsory features of their first sickle-cell programs. One reason for the repeals has been the response of blacks to the programs—our first genetic effort directed at a particular race. Although sickle-cell screening programs were introduced and supported by black legislators, the black response has been hostile. Robert Clark, a black Mississippi congressman who introduced a bill requiring the preschool testing of children for sickle-cell anemia, was told by some of his constituents, "White people are taking over the genetics of black people." James F. Bowman, director of laboratories at the University of Chicago, compared the new legislated genetics to "the racist eugenics legislation that led to the final solution in Nazi Germany." Others viewed sickle-cell screening as "racist genocide."

In an attempt to resolve some of the disagreement regarding the problem, the National Academy of Science's National Research Council (NAS–NRC) was asked to make suggestions for "wise, rational, and medically sound" guide-lines to screen and manage the sickle-cell-trait carriers in the armed forces. After a thorough review of the world's literature on the subject, the nine-member committee concluded: "There is insufficient scientific information to form a basis for exclud-ing them [people with the trait] from the armed forces or for limiting their activities or duties."

Within a month of publication of this study in mid-1973, United Air Lines responded by becoming the first airline in the United States to allow people with sickle-cell trait to hold cabin-attendant positions. Dr. George J. Kidera, vice president of medical services for the airline, explained it this way: "Sickle-cell anemia (the disease) and sickle-cell trait are, in fact, mutually exclusive, and the approximately two million blacks in the United States with sickle-cell trait should not be denied positions on the grounds that they have an incapacitat-ing disease—they do not."

But genetic myths die hard. In July 1973, Rodney Vessels reported for an ill-fated stint at the United States Air Force Academy. A black eighteen-year-old from King William County, Virginia, Vessels was setting out toward the fulfill-ment of a lifetime dream: to be the first black graduate of the

Air Force Academy. After less than a day, Rodney Vessels was sent home. Testing of his blood had revealed the genetic "disease" of sickle-cell trait.

Calling sickle-cell trait a "disease" and searching for chromosome indicators of criminality are only the latest in a series of genetic myths. Unless we're on the alert, the process can be repeated again and again. All that is required to create a genetic myth is the combination of an incorrect genetic conception (sickle-cell trait is a genetic disease) and its wholesale application (people with the trait shouldn't be allowed to work on airplanes). Of course this is nothing new. The misapplications of genetics in everyday American life have a long and colorful history. It all began with Francis Galton, the "father of modern eugenics." Galton, a tireless crusader for the improvement of the "race" in the nineteenth century, combined a scientist's curiosity with a missionary zeal for gaining national acceptance for his newly formulated science. "An enthusiasm to improve the race is so noble in its aim that it might well give rise to the sense of a religious obligation." So Galton enthused.

The major impulse leading to eugenics was a concern with preventing what was viewed at the time as the burden of human defect. Galton and his followers, the first eugenicists, attempted nothing less than the control, even prevention, of the propagation of the "unfit." They anchored their "science" on the newly discovered "rules" of criminal anthropology, which were simply a scientific version of the popular belief that criminals could be recognized by their appearance. According to Cesare Lombroso, the foremost "authority" in this field, every criminal type could be recognized by his distinguishing physical traits. Club feet, curvature of the spine, high-arched hard palate in the mouth—all were signs of "degeneration" that passed from parent to child. In one generation drunkenness might result from the "hereditary trait"; in another, epilepsy or insanity; two or three generations later, homicidal tendencies. Once the "bad seed" was present, nothing could eradicate it—nothing, that is, except the eugenic solution of preventing the "breeding" of those with the "genetic taint."

Galton focused on trying to establish compulsory means to limit the "breeding" of the insane, feebleminded, confined criminals, and paupers. In turn, he advocated that certificates of merit be given to young men and women showing favorable genetic traits. No less a figure than George Bernard Shaw became fired with enthusiam for all this. "There is now no reasonable excuse for refusing to face the fact that nothing but a eugenics religion can save our civilization from the fate that has overtaken all previous civilizations," Shaw proclaimed.

Further elaboration of eugenics theory, coupled with Galton's ceaseless appeal to the politicians and the journalists of the time, finally paid off. A villain was settled upon: the feebleminded. Drunkenness, insanity, laziness, criminality, sexual perversion—you name it—could be traced to feeblemindedness, what we refer to now as "mental retardation." The association of feeblemindedness with criminality and insanity took hold in state legislatures across the country. "What right had we to permit them [the children] to be born of parents who were depraved in body and mind?" asked Josephine Shaw Lowell, the first woman member of the New York State Board of Charities in 1877. And in "Feeblemindedness as an Inheritance," Ernest Bicknell estimated the cost accounting of feeblemindedness: "It is impossible to calculate what even one feebleminded woman may cost the public when her vast possibilities for evil as a producer of paupers and criminals through an endless line of descendants is considered."

Practical applications of the new theory were not long in coming. New Jersey has the dubious honor of opening the first asylum to confine the feebleminded, thus "containing the hereditary taint of feeblemindedness." More active measures soon followed. Dr. F. Hoyt Pilcher, superintendent of the Kansas State Home for the Feebleminded, published an account in the late 1890s of successful castration of forty-four feebleminded boys. When a public outcry erupted in the community in response to Pilcher's article, a reply by the Board of Trustees of the Home came quickly to the point: "Those who are now criticizing Dr. Pilcher will in a few years be talking of creating a monument to his memory."

The word was out. Feeblemindedness was the problem, castration and confinement the solution. In 1907, Indiana passed a bill making mandatory the sterilization of idiots, imbeciles, and the feebleminded. Eugenic marriage laws followed: "No man or woman either of whom is epileptic or imbecile or feebleminded shall marry or have extramarital relations," according to a statute in Connecticut, the first state to regulate marriage for "breeding purposes." Rhapsodic accounts followed in the scientific literature of the beneficial results of applied eugenics. Here is one by a Dr. Barr written in 1905: "One of the benefitees was a sexual pervert of the most pronounced description who would salute women on the road and was extremely vulgar in every way . . . and is now languid in movement and has developed a most excellent soprano singing voice and has improved in temper and habits."

Dr. Harry Sharpe, who introduced vasectomy in the United States in 1899, tried vasectomy on a nineteen-year-old inmate of the Indiana Reformatory who masturbated "over ten times a day." When the results were sufficiently spectacular, Sharpe wrote, "It was then that it occurred to me that this would be a good method of preventing procreation in the defectives and physically unfit."

By the turn of the century the sterilization of "idiots" and "imbeciles" had become standard procedure in many of the nation's mental hospitals. The legalities of these procedures, however, had never been adequately defined. In 1924 the issue reached the Supreme Court, where the proponents of eugenic sterilization achieved a decisive victory in the case of *Buck* v. *Bell*.

The plaintiff, Carrie Buck, was, according to the opinion of the court as written by Chief Justice Oliver Wendell Holmes, "a feebleminded white woman" committed to the Virginia State Colony for Epileptics and Feebleminded. "She is the daughter of a feebleminded mother in the same institution and the mother of an illegitimate feebleminded child," Holmes wrote.

Shortly after her admission at age eighteen to the State Colony, a Virginia law was passed which stated that "the health of the patient and the welfare of society may be promoted in certain cases by the sterilization of mental defectives." The act was contested in a suit brought against J. H. Bell, superintendent of the State Colony, alleging that the act of the Virginia Assembly denied Carrie Buck the equal protection of the law granted by the Fourteenth Amendment.

Chief Justice Holmes's summation of the case included the following remarks: "We have seen more than once that the public welfare may call upon the best citizens for their lives. It would be strange if we could not call upon those who already sap the strength of the state for these lesser sacrifices, often not felt to be such by those concerned, in order to prevent our being swamped with incompetence. It is better for the world if instead of waiting to execute degenerate offspring for crime, or let them starve from imbecility, society can prevent those who are manifestly unfit from continuing their kind. The principle that sustains compulsory vaccination is broad enough to cover cutting the fallopian tubes. *Three generations of imbeciles are enough.*"

Looking back fifty years later, it is startling to realize that nothing in the way of scientific proof was ever produced to justify these extreme measures. The genetic myth that feeblemindedness passed from generation to generation and got worse as it went along was self-perpetuating. Once it was accepted that feeblemindedness bred criminality and insanity and, in addition, cost everybody else money and trouble, the door swung wide open for increasingly extreme and grandiose measures to stamp it out.

In the years since *Buck* v. *Bell* the Pilchers and Galtons and Sharpes have faded into the pages of a pathetic and regrettable history; eugenics has become synonymous with racism and totalitarianism. But are the XYY and the sickle-cell-trait "myths" any less eugenic in scope, with their emphasis on the elimination of "criminality" and "the improvement of a race"? Are we now on the threshold of a new era of genetic peril?

As of this writing, the XYY and the sickle-cell-trait hullabaloos are finally settling down. Men with XYY chromosomes need no longer cower in fear when reporting for their annual company physicals; blacks can now work on airlines and will probably even be able to get into the Air Force Academy again. But what other genetic "diseases" are waiting in the wings to throw a mantle of scientific respectability over new and socially destructive myths? Can genetics be used again in the service of exploitation and racial prejudice?

Some Proposals

To draw any conclusions at this point regarding the controversies inherent in issues as complex as embryo transfer or AID or the goals and limitations of genetic screening would be simplistic and premature. As I mentioned at the beginning of this book, there may be no right or wrong answers. Instead, the choices may lie between alternative courses of action that will result in bringing us closer to the kind of society we want to live in over the next thirty or fifty years. If notions such as the "family" or "genetic identity" seem not worth preserving, then something like the additional and anonymous artificial insemination banks now being planned should pose no problems. The crucial point is that we realize as clearly as possible the implications of the choices we are making when we encourage certain biomedical technologies at the expense of others.

My research during the last two years has suggested to me a basic list of arguable propositions. They are not answers, but they suggest the means of arriving at answers. (Throughout, I have tried to identify my own prejudices and beliefs so as not to force them on anyone else as the right or correct answers. I hope I have been successful.) Rational and meaningful public policy decisions could be developed by public concern and debate along these lines. I believe almost any *choice* is preferable to the present condition—with unrestrained and directionless genetic biotechnology developing in the absence of any policy at all.

■   First, the traditional approach, using whatever biotechnology is available without reference to its social consequences, is irresponsible and can no longer be tolerated. The scientist's tendency to ivory-towerism must be countered by sober, everyday evaluations by public policy makers as to how scientific research will affect the quality of our lives. (In the last part of this book I suggest some of the ways these evaluations could be carried out.)

■   The prevailing concept of "genetic health" is a meaningless one. How can anyone be considered genetically healthy when we all carry a small but definite number of lethal genes? "Genetic health" in any absolute sense is another myth. No one is completely healthy any more than anyone is completely good. Now we seem hell-bent on achieving a genetic ideal where nobody will be the potential inheritor of a "disease," perhaps defined as narrowly as "susceptibility" to asthma, say, or even to dental caries. This is unreasonable. Even if gene therapies were to become a reality within twenty years, the mutation rate will guarantee that corrections of genetic defects will be counterbalanced by new and unpredictable genetic mutations. For one thing, all of us are exposed to unprecedented amounts of radiation, and we ingest mind-boggling numbers of chemicals in our food. The effects of these agents will not be known until late in our own lifetime. Ironically, we may be in for more rather than less genetic disease, an overall reduction rather than an increase in national "genetic health."

■   Applied genetics will always exert an almost quasi-mystical fascination for those predisposed to tyranny and theories of racial superiority. Another eugenics movement can arise at any time. In fact, thanks to Professors Arthur Jensen and Richard Herrnstein, we are presently experiencing a renaissance of the ancient theory that Caucasians are more intelligent than blacks or those from the Third World. Once again a "scientific" issue is debated without reference to the fact that the worst brutalities and inhumanities have been performed in the interest of developing a "pure race" or in the assertion of genetic superiority.

■ The genetic contribution to physical and mental characteristics is a large one, and the implications of this must be faced. For years we have emphasized the importance of environment in the development of physical and mental diseases. Now studies are providing us with proof that genes are critical determinants in an increasing number of physical and mental diseases, and to all indications the list of such diseases will grow. Like it or not, biomedical technology is soon going to tell us more about our physical and mental health than some of us may care to know. We cannot deny this reality by continuing to overemphasize the importance of the environment. Artificial insemination using anonymous sperm donors in this modern context is unscientific and deprives the person born from this procedure of a distinct identity. Imagine for a moment knowing absolutely nothing about your father, not even from your mother, who doesn't know who he is either. A small number of people endure this situation now. But do we wish to increase that number? Closely allied to this is the issue of embryo transfer. Should this be evaluated only in reference to the "suffering" of infertile couples? Might this not have a potential for dehumanizing one of the most personal aspects of our lives? As long as there have been forms of contraception, we've had sex without procreation. What will be the effect of procreation without sex?

■ Screening programs for the purpose of "controlling" genetic "disease" or its carriers are fraught with medical and racial myths that can be deeply divisive and explosive. Decisions regarding which genetic diseases will be the object of future screening and research are not, and should no longer be considered, as strictly medical ones. Behind the encouragement and funding of certain lines of research you can discover a whole set of attitudes and social preconceptions. Sometimes, as with sickle-cell anemia, the preconceptions are obvious: "Don't ask for volunteers for screening; don't make voluntary programs available. Rather, *those people* have to undergo testing; the programs have to be mandatory." In other instances the "loading" of preconceptions is harder to see. Take lead poisoning, which occurs almost exclusively in the ghettos. Programs should be set up that do justice to the social complexities of why ghetto kids eat the paint off their walls and not be confined to the treatment of those already poisoned. Preventive medicine must concern itself with more than just *medicine*.

■　　The genetic counselor has only one duty—to his patient or client. All other responsibilities, to "society" or to the "next generation," are secondary. In genetic counseling and prenatal diagnosis, the counselor must clearly distinguish his personal moral, religious, and ethical beliefs from the advice that he offers. Once again, strict reliance on the medical frame of reference is distorted and confining. In my visits to genetic clinics across the country, I've been impressed with the pomposity and self-righteousness of many genetic counselors. Rather than envisioning their business as principally educative, many of them are quick to foist their own value judgments on the people coming to them for help. Since the typical counselor is a member of the middle class, his clients end up with a suburban-trimmed-lawn-private-school notion of what sort of children they should have.

■　　A purpose would be served by dividing different emerging genetic technologies into classifications of low, intermediate, and high potential for social and ethical conflict. One of the most basic divisions concerns the immediacy of certain developments. For example, in the last three years innumerable articles have appeared regarding cloning. One would think the cloned man was just around the corner. Yet in my research and interviews I failed to find even one genetic authority who would fix the achievement of human cloning at less than twenty years. Clearly much more immediate issues demand our attention than cloning.

Closely allied to this is the tendency of some geneticists to arrogate to themselves the role of "engineers" of the next generation. Using presently developed technology (screening, amniocentesis, selective abortion), they are well on the way toward convincing us that we have an absolute right to *perfectly* healthy children. I believe the right to have healthy children is relative; it does not justify the use of technology for obtaining such inconsequential things as eye color, for instance. To select and reject human beings by the consumer criteria of the marketplace lessens the humanity of us all.

■ A moratorium is in order on human research on *in vitro* fertilization until further animal work has been done and standards on human experimentation have been established. The latest National Institutes of Health guideline on human research has written in it just such a moratorium on fetal research.

■ "Informed consent" should be the foundation on which to judge genetic research. When "informed consent" is not possible, the research is unethical and dehumanizing. This ultimately rules out certain types of research on the very young and on those who for one reason or another cannot be made to understand the possible consequences of research.

■ It is reasonable for us to develop and use technology directed toward the cure of presently fatal and seriously disabling genetic diseases. But goals concerning such things as increasing the intelligence of future generations are inappropriate and eugenic in character.

■ Decisions regarding the encouragement and funding of genetic technologies are public ones and should be made by all of us, not just by elitist "institutes" and "centers" where the poor, the inarticulate, and the uneducated have no influence. During my visits to several existing bioethical institutes I was impressed with the depth of scholarly research done by their members. Unfortunately some of them did not think it necessary to draw on the opinions of those with experience and qualifications outside traditional "academic" circles. Unfortunately again, whatever attention the government is now giving to the biotechnological issues is being funneled through these institutes via advisory panels, reports, etc. As I explain in the last part of this book, I favor an increased democratization of the decision-making processes regarding biomedical technology. There is no place for intellectual elitism in areas that concern all of us so intimately. One Manhattan Project in any generation is one too many.

This forms only a bare-bones' outline for the development of a genetic biomedical technology we can live with. Some of the people to whom I have showed these propositions have disagreed violently with them. That is why I've called them *arguable*. Out of debate, even argument, can come meaningful choice. But whatever biomedical technology we finally choose, and choose we must, perhaps even by default, our greatest challenge remains the formulation of a code for human experimentation.

The essence of any science is experimentation: the pitting of the best in available talent and technical resources in the service of achieving meaningful scientific breakthroughs. Despite two hundred years of human experimentation, however, any organized attempt to regulate and define the allowable limits dates back no more than twenty-five years. The story of the development of controls in human experimentation, while strikingly contemporary, is also filled with the worst examples of cruelty, injustice, greed, and the triumph of special-interest considerations. As I show in the next section, very little has changed over the years; a just formulation regulating human experimentation will not be easy to come by.

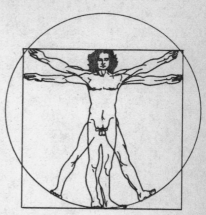

Part Three

The Animal of Necessity

A Game of
Russian Roulette

*In a game of Russian roulette
an unfortunate result cannot be
regarded as unpredictable.*
      —VERNON G. CAVE

One day in 1932, Charles Wesley Pollard turned up for the first in a series of injections that he would continue to receive during the next twenty-five years. A black farm worker in rural Alabama, Pollard, together with some four hundred other black men, was told after his blood was tested that he had "bad blood" and would require "shots" for an indefinite period. Over the years, Pollard and the others reported on command to a schoolhouse near the tiny town of Shiloh, where, in the absence of a clinic or physician's office, the nicknamed "606" shots were administered under an oak tree in the school playground. At the completion of their "treatment," each of the men received $25 and a certificate: "U.S. Public Health Service. This certificate is awarded in grateful recognition of twenty-five years of participation in the Tuskegee Medical Research Study."

In the summer of 1972 Pollard read in the *Birmingham News* an article about "the Tuskegee syphilis study," but he did not connect it with his series of shots. Previously a reporter had questioned him about the injections, and he had not had much to say. But suddenly the pieces began to fit together: Pollard and four hundred others had been unknowing subjects in a ghastly experiment where "treatment" had not been treatment at all but a morbidly prolonged observation period of the overall effects of untreated syphilis on physical and mental health.

As just about everybody knows these days, syphilis is a venereal disease traceable to a microscopic organism—the spirochete. Smears prepared from a fresh syphilitic lesion, when studied under a microscope, are seen to contain vast numbers of the specially fluorescing spirochetes. In a short time, with or without treatment, the syphilitic lesion disappears; along with it disappears the chance for a quick and easy diagnosis. Soon the signs and symptoms are too vague even for skilled physicians to spot; they may well overlook the possibility of syphilis as they sort through a maze of varying complaints. The diagnostic clues eventually become so nonspecific that the only way to diagnose syphilis with close to 100 per cent accuracy is to test the blood and spinal fluid for positive confirmation of the disease. Diagnosis is critical, however, since an efficient treatment exists: penicillin or other antibiotics. If syphilis can be diagnosed and treated early enough, it can be eliminated completely. All of which has caused scientists to wonder through the years: "What happens to the untreated cases? What is the natural history of the disease?" It fell to Charles Wesley Pollard and four hundred other black men who suffered from syphilis to find this out for us.

By 1936, four years after the start of the study, the first of the Tuskegee reports appeared comparing the men receiving genuine treatment with those receiving placebos. The rates of illness were these: 84 per cent of the untreated were ill in some way, compared to only 39 per cent in the treated groups. (It must be remembered that penicillin was not in general use until the early 1950s.) By 1942, when the study was ten years old, the death rate for the untreated was 24.6 per cent, compared to 13.9 per cent among the treated. By 1952, 40 per cent of those who had received no treatment were dead, compared to 20 per cent among the treated. In every category of ailment—death, heart disease, nervous-system involvement, bone disease—the group with untreated syphilis significantly outnumbered those who had been given medication. But the study continued; even today, some of the men have not yet heard that their "treatment" was a sham. No effort was made to halt the research until 1966; at that time a public health adviser, Peter Buxton, wrote to the chief of the Venereal Disease Program at the National Communicable Disease Center. His letter was never answered. Finally, in 1972, in a series of articles by Jean Heller of the Associated Press, the Tuskegee syphilis study was brought to public attention. On August 28 an ad hoc advisory panel appointed by the Department of Health, Education, and Welfare began an investigation. The nine-member panel—citizens drawn from medicine, law, the church, labor, education, health administration, and public affairs—began looking into the history of the Tuskegee study.

From the start, the panel's attempts to locate any written protocols of the Tuskegee study turned up nothing. No protocol was ever produced documenting the original intent of the study. Even in 1936, when the first report appeared, no statement was made as to the goal, except for one grim memorandum: "Plans for the continuation of this study are under way. During the past 12 months success has been obtained in gaining permission for the performance of autopsies on 11 of 15 individuals who died." The purpose seems to have been to document what would happen to untreated patients with syphilis. As one of the senior investigators wrote, "Since a considerable portion of the infected Negro population remained untreated during the entire course of syphilis . . . an unusual opportunity [arose] to study the untreated syphilitic patient from the beginning of the disease to the death of the infected persons." No reference was made to the central fact that by the late 1940s a specific drug, penicillin, existed to cure syphilis and *was being deliberately withheld* in the interests of the study. None of the participants was informed of the nature of their disease or given the opportunity to choose or not choose treatment. "The United States Public Health Service from the onset of the study maintained a continuous policy of withholding treatment for syphilis from the infected subjects," said the panel's report. Yet a technical and advisory group, convened in 1969 by the Health Service, concluded that little medical knowledge had been gained from the study. Despite this, no recommendation was made to terminate it; instead, the group recommended "with some ambiguity that the participants surviving at that time should not be treated."

In a final report of April 1973 the Tuskegee panel published its findings: (1) In retrospect, the Public Health Service Study of Untreated Syphilis in the Male Negro in Macon County, Alabama, was ethically unjustified in 1932. (2)

The study should be terminated immediately. (3) "No uniform departmental policy for the protection of research subjects exists."

In a very real sense, another Tuskegee could occur at any time. As an isolated phenomenon, the Tuskegee study would be bad enough. But, in the words of the panel, "The Tuskegee Syphilis Study, placed in the perspective of its early years, is not an isolated event in the terms of the generally accepted conditions and practices that prevailed in the 1930s."

Such "generally accepted conditions and practices" are not limited to the 1930s. Consider a more recent example of human experimentation:

Willowbrook, located on Staten Island, in New York, is a large complex of twenty-four buildings that house mentally retarded children. Most of the children—they total about five thousand—are between the ages of three and ten. In 1949 the incidence of hepatitis among these children began to climb alarmingly. Soon it became clear that the spread of the disease was out of control; many children showed only the mildest of symptoms but nevertheless suffered severe liver damage. Moreover, no method of control could be devised, for overcrowding and primitive sanitary conditions contributed to a rapid, sometimes explosive spread of the infection.

In 1956 a study sponsored by the Armed Forces Epidemiologic Board and endorsed by the executive faculty of New York University School of Medicine, set out to develop a vaccine against hepatitis. The crux of the experiment involved the administration of live hepatitis virus to some of the mentally retarded children at Willowbrook. The justification for this experiment went roughly like this: Most of the children were going to contract hepatitis at some point in their stay at Willowbrook anyway. Many of these would not be diagnosed if the case were mild, even if it resulted in severe liver damage. By deliberately giving the hepatitis virus, an extremely mild form of the infection would be induced, followed by immunity. In the event that hepatitis developed, the children would be under care in a special, well-equipped, optimally staffed unit.

From this study came the most definitive documentation ever accomplished of two different forms of hepatitis—

THE ANIMAL OF NECESSITY

MS1 strain and MS2 strain. Each differs in terms of the incubation period required for the disease to develop and, more importantly, in the immunity conferred: children infected with either of the virus strains become resistant to subsequent attempts at infection by the same virus strain. By almost any scientific parameter, the study was a success, and the results were published in such prestigious journals as the *Journal of the American Medical Association* and the *New England Journal of Medicine*.

The Willowbrook experiment, as with the "606" shots given to Charles Wesley Pollard, demonstrates the morally numbing effect that medical jargon seems to exert on some experimenters. Behind the verbal neutrality of "control groups" and "incubation periods" lurked a potential for horror which the researchers either didn't see or chose to ignore—like rapt spectators in an art gallery grimly tuning out the gruesome sound of a child's fall from a balustrade. As all the researchers knew, hepatitis has a wide range of severity and can be fatal; and it cannot always be controlled even with the best medical care. In addition, the arguments used to justify the study revolved around social rather than medical conditions. If hepatitis was rampant at Willowbrook because of its crowded and unsanitary conditions, was the development of a new vaccine an appropriate solution? Why not clean up and clear out Willowbrook? Perhaps what was called for was a full-scale revision of the prevailing attitude at the time about the care of the mentally retarded. To make things worse, all existing medical measures to eliminate hepatitis at Willowbrook had not yet been exhausted. Ironically, the same group conducting the experiment had written, ten years earlier, of the effectiveness of immune gamma globulin in the treatment of hepatitis (resulting in a reduction of 85 per cent in MS1 hepatitis). But gamma globulin was not used on the children at Willowbrook. In summary, a situation existed where a potentially lethal virus was deliberately introduced to retarded children and an acceptable method of medical treatment withheld in the interest of the experiment.

There is every reason to believe that Willowbrook would never have come to public attention were it not for the efforts of Dr. Henry K. Beecher, professor of anesthesiology at Harvard Medical School. In 1966 Dr. Beecher wrote an article in the *New England Journal of Medicine* on the ethics of clinical research. In his article Dr. Beecher described twenty-two published experiments which he considered medically unethical. Among the twenty-two examples was Willowbrook. Quoting from the World Medical Association's Draft Code of Ethics on Human Experimentation, Dr. Beecher concluded: "Any act or advice which could weaken physical or mental resistance of a human being may be used only in his interest." As Dr. Beecher pointed out, the administration of a potentially lethal virus to helpless children could not possibly be acceptable under the World Medical Association guidelines.

The response to Dr. Beecher's article was explosive. In a series of letters to medical journals around the world, his fellow physicians questioned Dr. Beecher's integrity, his allegiance to medical customs, the reliability of his scholarship, even the motives behind his concern. In an unprecedented gesture, Dr. Franz Ingelfinger, editor of the *New England Journal of Medicine*, came to the defense of Dr. Saul Krugman, the Willowbrook experimenter: "How much better to have a patient with hepatitis, accidentally or deliberately acquired, under the guidance of a Krugman than under the care of a zealot who would exercise intuitive management, blind to the fact that his one-track efforts to protect the rights of the individual are in fact depriving that individual of his right to good medical care."

Others saw the issue in less glowing terms. The influential British medical journal *Lancet* editorialized that "the giving of infected material to children who would not directly benefit could not be justified." In response to this, Dr. Krugman repeated his assertion that in his judgment it is better to infect the children with hepatitis virus under the controlled circumstances of his special unit than for the children to be exposed to the same virus naturally under the less favorable conditions of Willowbrook's wards. The *Journal of the American Medical Association* congratulated Krugman and his coworkers on a contribution which would have been "impossible without the judicious use of human beings in carefully controlled experimental studies."

In early 1974 I contacted Dr. Ingelfinger to find out whether he had changed his mind regarding his favorable opinion of the Willowbrook study. He acknowledged that: "in the last seven years I have become more ambivalent and troubled" by the Willowbrook experiments; he found particularly troubling the "indications that parents were coerced to agree to the experiments by being told that admissions would be delayed unless they were willing to put their children on the experimental ward."

Despite such reservations, data from the Willowbrook experiments continue to be published in prestigious medical journals throughout the world, thus clearly demonstrating that no unified concept exists at this time that a medical experiment must be both scientifically valid and ethically justifiable. I believe the ultimate importance of the Willowbrook study has yet to be gauged. Its importance will be measured in the years to come by our response to this most outrageous assault on personal freedom and dignity. It will stand as a challenge to our traditional ideas concerning the limits of human experimentation.

What Man Has Done to Man

From my earliest experiences in medical school I have been struck with the differences between research and practicing physicians. The latter group—in which I include myself—is primarily interested in the care of individual patients one at a time, without any broader reference to "groups" or "populations." This approach, individual- and practice-oriented, has been dominated for years on the

American medical scene by the medical researchers for whom every patient is a means to achieve further "discoveries." I hope this does not sound like a slur on research doctors because it is not meant to be. Some of the finest doctors I've been privileged to encounter have conducted biomedical research with intelligence, wisdom, and compassion. Nevertheless, as a group, researchers march to a different drummer; individual patients are only a means to a much more ambitious end: the attainment of that academic recognition which is the reward of the successful researcher.

The actual day-to-day details of how experimenters carry out their experiments has, until recently, been of interest only to other scientists. Traditionally, their experimental methods have been described in the opening paragraphs of published scientific works, where any references to the people involved in the experiment have been carefully removed, leaving the reader with the eerie feeling that somehow the experimental subjects involved weren't *real people*. In an attempt to get beyond the scientific euphemisms, I made a search of the available literature on the history of human experimentation. I was not long at my task, however, until I discovered to my surprise that a good history of human experimentation has never been written. Isolated accounts exist, however, about how certain medical experiments were carried out. One curious and fascinating book is *Memoirs of a Physician* by Vikenty Verassayev, a Russian. Published in 1916 and long out of print, it is a sobering account of the early days of one aspect of human experimentation: the development of our modern ideas on venereal disease.

Today we are better informed than any previous generation in the details of venereal disease. The story of how we came by this knowledge is the subject of Verassayev's book. In the 1880s, when Verassayev began his narrative, a specific microorganism, the gonococcus, was isolated as the cause of gonorrhea. Absolute proof depended, however, on producing the disease in man by deliberate inoculations. This was ultimately accomplished in "a patient suffering from creeping paralysis whose death was awaited very shortly." The inoculation was judged "a brilliant success," according to the experi-

THE ANIMAL OF NECESSITY

menter, Dr. Max Bockhart, who found evidence on autopsy examination of "acute gonorrhea inflammation" in the bladder and lower urinary tract. Next, inoculations were given to a healthy man, resulting in gonococcal inflammation. The experimenter, Dr. Ernest Bunn, noted in passing that "acute gonorrheic infection is one of the most important causes of painful and serious affections of the sexual organs."

For years, gonorrhea had been postulated as a cause of inflammation in the eyes of newborn infants, resulting from exposure during birth to the gonococcus in the birth canal of an infected mother. Dr. E. Frankel inoculated the eyes of a sickly infant with secretions from gonorrhea patients and produced "typical purulent inflammation of the eyes."

Turning then to syphilis, a series of highly original investigators established for the first time the contagious nature of syphilitic skin lesions. Witness a typical experiment:

"First experiment: Durst, a boy of 12, registration number 1396, suffered for a number of years from sores on the head. Otherwise quite healthy. As his disease required detention in hospital for several months and as he had not suffered from syphilis in the past we found him to be very suitable for inoculation, which was performed on August 6. The skin of the right thigh was incised and the pus taken from a syphilitic patient introduced into the fresh and slightly bleeding wounds. I rubbed the matter into abrasions with a spatula, then I rubbed the scarified surface with lint soaked in the same matter, and having covered it with the same lint, applied a bandage. About the beginning of October the child developed a typical syphilitic rash."

Research such as that on Durst established once and for all the contagiousness of syphilitic skin lesions. Doubts still persisted, however, that syphilis, once cured, could be contracted again.

"M., 37, with paralysis of the lower extremities . . . had been cured of syphilis. . . . Wounds were dressed with lint soaked in matter taken from the mucous papules of another patient. . . . [Later] The wounds had become covered with a greyish membrane, suppuration very copious and of disgusting odor. Lint saturated with the same pus as previously was freshly applied to the wound." Pleased with these results, the experimenter, Professor Vidal de Cassi, chided his fellow researchers for their timidity. "Unfortunately the cleverest of syphilologists, who could be of the greatest service to science thanks to their logic and clinical observations, regard experiment as immoral and neglect it accordingly."

Verassayev's catalogue of horrors continues: the milk of a syphilitic woman injected under the skin of a ten-year-old prostitute; the pus from a syphilitic patient used to inoculate a leper; the secretion of syphilitic lesions from the breast of a wet nurse inoculated into a patient of fifty.

Turning to researchers on nonvenereal diseases, Verassayev's account included American researchers, with special reference to an experiment on preventive inoculation against scarlet fever. The researcher, a Dr. Stickler, observed that persons who had contracted certain diseases from farm animals often became immune to scarlet fever. To verify this, Stickler first injected children with the blood of sick horses and cows, then placed the children on sheets which had been used by scarlet-fever patients and made them inhale the air emanating from the sheets. Finally, he injected the blood of scarlet-fever patients into twenty children without producing a fatality. Inspired by these results, Dr. Stickler presented a summary of his work at the Academy of Medicine in New York. A commentary on his paper included: "The results obtained are, in any case, sufficiently important to encourage further research in the same direction."

Behind Verassayev's memoirs lies a piquant outrage and horror: "One thing is established beyond all vestige of a doubt—and that is the shameful indifference with which the medical world contemplates such atrocities." The memoirs, written decades before Willowbrook or Tuskegee, strike a chilling contemporary note. "The moment has arrived for society to take its own measures of self-protection against those zealots of science who have ceased to distinguish between their brothers and guinea pigs."

Until recently, the importance of protecting the treated against those administering the treatment—in essence, the protection of the patient against the doctor-researcher—

wasn't any more obvious than in Verassayev's day. In the popular view, doctors are supposed to cure the patient of his illness or, when a cure is not possible, at least to work toward the patient's comfort and well-being. Useful as this view may be in particular instances, it breaks down entirely when experimental treatments are compared to traditional ones. Here the dangerous and unproved are often substituted for accepted but often ineffective treatments. Or, as with Tuskegee and Willowbrook, traditional treatments are done away with altogether for the purpose of more precisely defining the disease under study.

The first measure to protect patients against "experiments" can be traced in English law to a court statement of 1767: "Many men very skillful in their profession have frequently acted out of the common way for the sake of trying experiments. They have acted ignorantly and unskillfully, contrary to the known rule and usage." At a later date, references can be found in the French literature warning of the dangers of having human subjects in experimental medical procedures. By 1883 an American researcher, William Beaumont, commented on sound scientific principles as a protection for the patient. Beyond these few instances, however, there exists very little in the way of protection for subjects in human experiments. Those that do exist owe their origins to the Nazi prison camp "experiments."

By 1945 (the midway point of the Tuskegee study), a tribunal of distinguished American and European jurists drew up the Nuremberg Code; this was a response to the information gained at Nuremberg about Nazi physicians in concentration camps who had conducted medical experiments without any regard for human life. It remains an often quoted authority for what is and is not allowable in human experimentation. Ironically, panels of American scientists testified at the Nuremberg trials that abuses similar to the Nazis' could not occur in the United States. This at the same time when men in Tuskegee were being injected with placebos against a disease that was slowly tearing up their aortas and wreaking silent devastation throughout their bodies.

At the conclusion of the Nazi physicians' trial, the

Military Tribunal of Nuremberg set down ten basic principles for human experimentation. In essence, these are the principles of the Nuremberg Code:

1.   The voluntary consent of the human subject is absolutely essential.

2.   The experiment should be such as to yield fruitful results for the good of society, unprocurable by other methods or means of study, and not random or unnecessary in nature.

3.   The experiment should be so designed and based on the results of animal experimentation and a knowledge of the natural history of the disease or other problems under study that the anticipated results will justify the performance of the experiment.

4.   The experiment should be so conducted as to avoid all unnecessary physical and mental suffering and injury.

5.   No experiment should be conducted where there is a prior reason to believe that death or disabling injury will occur; except, perhaps, in those experiments where the experimental physicians also serve as subject.

6.   The degree of risk to be taken should never exceed that determined by the humanitarian importance of the problem to be solved by the experiment.

7.   Proper preparations should be made and adequate facilities provided to protect the experimental subject against even remote possibility of injury, disability, or death.

8.   The experiment should be conducted only by scientifically qualified persons. The highest degree of skill and care should be required through all stages of the experiment of those who conduct or engage in the experiment.

9.   During the course of the experiment the human subject should be at liberty to bring the experiment to an end if he has reached the physical or mental state where the continuation of the experiment seems to him impossible.

10.   During the course of the experiment the scientist in charge must be prepared to terminate the experiment at any stage if he has probable cause to believe, in the exercise of the good faith, superior skill, and careful judgment required of

him, that a continuation of the experiment is likely to result in injury, disability, or death of the experimental subject.

In the almost thirty years since the drafting of the Nuremberg Code, no less than thirty-eight other codes have been developed to make up for its shortcomings. Despite differences in emphasis and wording, all rely on self-regulation by the investigators. All are variations on the theme that research investigators can be handed a sort of Ten Commandments which they will voluntarily obey in their own research investigations. But one important consideration is ignored in all of these codes: the personalities of the medical researchers.

Monsters or Saints?

Until recently, most studies about medical research scientists were anecdotal and impressionistic. If you were convinced that experimenters were monsters, books such as Verassayev's provided data to support that conclusion. Alternately, medical history could provide instances of almost sainted altruism, such as Walter Reed's experimental studies combating yellow fever. Both the "monster" theory and the "saint" theory were based on stereotypes. In 1969 Bernard Barber, a sociologist at Columbia University, began the first study on medical researchers that substituted hard data for impressions or stereotypes.

Over three years Professor Barber interviewed 350 research physicians involved in 424 different studies that used human subjects. Under conditions of stringent confidentiality, he asked the researchers to estimate how much benefit resulted from their studies, how much risk there was for the subjects, the possible benefit for future patients, and, finally, the scientific value of the research projects. Tabulation of results indicated that 18 per cent of the studies involved more risk than benefit for the patients participating in the research. With these data, Professor Barber and his co-workers dug a little deeper, inquiring into the type of patient selected for human experimentation. "We found that studies where the risks are relatively high, in proportion to the therapeutic benefits for the subjects, are almost twice as likely to use subjects more than three-fourths of whom are ward or clinic patients." The poor, the retarded, the imprisoned, the chronically hospitalized—Professor Barber found the large majority of subjects for human experimentation drawn from these groups. "Even when we put the benefits to future patients and possible benefit to medical knowledge in the balance, we still found that the least favorable studies were almost twice as likely to be done on ward or clinic patients."

In the second part of his book, *Research on Human Subjects: Problems of Social Control on Medical Experimentation,* Professor Barber concentrates on an issue even closer to the bone: the ethical values of those presently engaged in biomedical research.

First, he investigated the researchers' own evaluations of priorities. Three hundred fifty researchers were asked to name three characteristics they most valued in potential research collaborators. Scientific ability was mentioned by 86 per cent; 45 per cent opted for "hard work"; "personality" was paramount to 45 per cent. When it came to the category "ethical concern for research subjects," only 6 per cent thought this important enough to even mention.

"When the researchers were confronted with this rather astounding data, several of those polled responded, 'Oh, I take ethical concern for granted.' Well, I don't take it so much for granted!" exclaims Barber.

Within two years of its publication, Barber's book was established as the most quoted source on the bioethics of human research. Its reception among the medical researchers themselves, however, has been about as cheery as that given an Internal Revenue Service audit. The usual response has been one of unstudied neglect. The *Journal of the American Medical*

Association, our most widely read medical journal, has not seen fit to review it.

Hearing Professor Barber speak at the hearings of the Senate Subcommittee on Health in July 1973, I was impressed with his intellectual vigor and his ability to discuss the most sobering issues with disarming candor. Tall, with thick, wavy white hair, and a sometimes startlingly piquant humor, Professor Barber is unique among bioethicists: clearly not for him are the somber doomsday tones that are now fashionable among his peers.

"In the past," he said, "compassion in the scientific investigator has been relied on as a sound basis for regulating human experimentation. I set out to measure just how sound this basis was." To test the hypothesis, Barber and a colleague, John J. Lally of Lehman College, set up a hypothetical experiment of their own: a hypothetical research proposal drawn up with the skilled help of practicing biomedical researchers. The proposed "study" involved the effect of radioactive calcium on bone metabolism in children suffering from a serious bone disease. As presented to the researchers, the "study," if successful, might eventually benefit the experimental group of children suffering from the disease; but it would have no benefit for a control group of healthy normal children. Finally, and most importantly, it would slightly increase the possibility of contracting leukemia for both the diseased *and the healthy* children.

"It seemed reasonable that a compassionate researcher would not subject healthy subjects to a study that could potentially increase their chances of later developing a disease as serious as leukemia," Professor Barber said. But over 46 per cent of the researchers he queried accepted his hypothetical research proposal, and 14 per cent would have approved the study even if the chances of success were as slim as one in ten! "Thus at least a significant minority of investigators does not seem to hold the standards of compassion and concern for subjects which are expected of them professionally."

Next Professor Barber tried to pin down those factors which increase or decrease the degree of the researcher's concern for his subjects. He started with a simple question: "Have you ever found yourself becoming involved emotionally with the people serving as subjects in your research to an extent greater than you deem desirable for a researcher?" Only 17 per cent of the physician-investigators responding answered yes.

"The response to this question was startling but consistent with what I have called the dilemma of science and therapy. In a very real sense a scientific investigator is facing a role conflict. As a physician, the doctor who is also a clinical investigator, with the obligation to be a scientist striving to advance knowledge through original discovery, is still bound by the obligation of concern for and compassionate care of those entrusted to him. How this role conflict is resolved was my next interest."

Very little previous investigation had been done on this knotty problem. Ironically, the one published source had been written fifteen years earlier by one of Barber's students, Renée Fox. In *Experiment Perilous*, Fox had discovered many instances of unusually close relationships between research physicians and patient subjects. This seemed to conflict with Barber's finding that only 17 per cent reported *ever* becoming involved emotionally with their subjects. "From this I thought it reasonable to assume that certain factors existed which tended to encourage or discourage compassion. I called these concern-producing factors and set out to describe them."

After months of painstaking analysis of his interview data, Barber arrived at a profile of "concern-producing factors." First, he found that more frequent and more personal interaction over a longer period of time tended to promote greater concern and involvement. Conversely, the doctors who were most removed from the day-to-day care of their research patients were the least compassionate. Second, involvement and concern tended to be stimulated when the studies involved procedures that were dangerous and painful, such as open-heart surgery. Finally, whenever a physician was both the investigator and the treating doctor, his degree of concern for his patients increased. When one person filled both roles, Barber noted an intensification of the science-therapy dilemma, often resulting in greater investigator involvement and concern. In such a situation the patient and doctor were not separated from each other by scientific protocol and laboratory mumbo jumbo.

Applying these findings, Barber was usually able to distinguish experiments likely to produce high investigator "concern" from those likely to be marked by a relative lack of "concern" on the part of the investigating doctor. For the most part, "concern" seemed more a result of the conditions of the experiment—contact with the subjects through day-to-day general medical management—than it did with any internal reserves, i.e., "compassion."

"The implications of this are critically important," according to Professor Barber. "The individual physician's capacity for compassion is just not sound enough for everybody's protection. More important is building concern-producing conditions into biomedical clinical research. Now the overall incidence of the conditions is far from universal. Instead, for the most part, they seem to occur relatively infrequently. In fact, there is some evidence, although we did not collect it systematically, that there are mechanisms which, whether intended or not, serve to protect clinical researchers from emotional involvement with subjects."

Although Professor Barber's point is that biomedical research serves to isolate the subjects from the researchers, he hastens to add that the "system" is not that way by design. "We're faced with a whole structural system based on ignorance. Because the emphasis has always been on the results of research rather than the quality of research methods, we're only just now starting to develop some guidelines. One thing seems pretty clear, however: in many ways medicine is too important to be left to the doctors; science is too important to be left to the scientists; and biomedical research is too important to be left to the biomedical researchers. Things cannot be left to go on as they have. Something must be done about human experimentation *now*."

One of the most articulate writers on human experimentation today is Dr. Jay Katz, a physician and a member of the faculty of the Yale University Law School. As a result of his experiences as a member of the

Tuskegee panel, Dr. Katz is also convinced that regulations are urgently needed on human experimentation: "The conscious and unconscious denial of widespread transgressions has many roots. . . . Suffice to say that the research community has made no concerted efforts either to improve any meaningful self-regulation on its practices or to discuss in any scholarly depth the permissible limits of human research. Regulation has to come from somewhere." But, Dr. Katz adds: "All existing judicial efforts have been riddled with loopholes and unanswered questions, nor can encouragement be expected from its members of the medical community. Professionals don't like regulations. They would like to do things the way they have been accustomed to doing them. They are afraid, in part, of facing up to troublesome questions about the research subject's rights."

The possessor of the reasoning powers of a logician, the affability of a professional diplomat, and a heavy German accent, Dr. Katz comes across as a kind of biomedical version of Henry Kissinger. During a meeting in his office on the second floor of the Yale University Law School, Katz outlined some of the problems. "It's really very basic," he says. "Most researchers on human subjects are poorly trained in terms of *talking with people.* Their medical education has not prepared them for interacting in a human way with their patients. One obstacle is the investigator's anxiety when he has to confront a subject with an open invitation to participate in a research enterprise."

Dr. Katz thinks it would be ideal if a researcher thought beforehand of the consequences of what he asks of his subject. " 'What am I asking the patient to go through? Should I or should I not ask him?' These confrontations with oneself and one's patient-subject are difficult, but they must be engaged in. Failing in this, as most researchers do, it's understandable why they cannot explain the risks sufficiently to obtain informed consent."

A lot of attention has been focused recently on informed consent as the basic issue in human experimentation. Although everybody thinks he knows what constitutes informed consent, Dr. Katz has discovered significant differences. "Consider six recently described elements of informed consent: A full explanation of the procedures to be followed, including an identification of those which are experimental; a description of the attendant discomforts and risks; a description of the benefits to be expected; a disclosure of appropriate alternative procedures that would be advantageous for the subject; an offer to answer any inquiries concerning the procedures; an instruction that the subject is free to withdraw his consent and to discontinue participation in the project or activity at any time. Looking at these elements of informed consent, you would assume unanimity existed. Yet another set of guidelines by the Public Health Service on informed consent totally omits the elements concerning disclosure of alternative procedures and an offer to answer inquiries concerning the procedures. Why have these been omitted? Obviously unanimity does *not* exist regarding 'informed consent.'"

To make things even more complicated, several studies point to the difficulties involved in obtaining informed consent. Some of them, in fact, suggest that informed consent may be impossible in certain clinical situations. In 1970 Drs. Carl Fellner and John Marshall studied the consent issue as it applied to kidney donors. Both anticipated that the decisions regarding kidney donation would be long and anguishing ones, marked by ambivalence and prolonged soul-searching. Instead, much to their surprise, the decision for or against donating a kidney was made at the time of the first contact with the kidney transplant team, often via a telephone conversation and long before the detailed information needed for "informed consent" was even provided. In a sense the decision was whimsical, even irrational. The investigators observed, "All the donors and potential donors reported a decision-making process that was immediate and 'irrational' and could not be accepted as an 'informed consent.' Actually, the medical renal-transplant teams did not permit these donors to volunteer until a prolonged process of repeated information had been completed. The effectiveness of the procedure must, however, be questioned . . . if for no other reason than that it did not dissuade one single volunteer."

In another study, a psychiatric profile was drawn up

on paid "normal" volunteers for a hallucinogenic drug study. The range and severity of psychopathology found were far in excess of what would be expected from any random sample where the degree of psychopathology would roughly equal that found in the general population. Obviously, the nature of the study to a large part determined the type of "normals" volunteering. "Informed consent" had nothing to do with their decision to volunteer, nor did it subsequently influence the decision in any way.

A lot of this could be avoided, according to Dr. Katz, by inviting nonscientists to participate in the conduct of scientific research. "The necessity of engaging nonscientists in the evaluation of research is comparatively new and has special significance when we talk about informed consent. It has been insufficiently recognized that the decision to conduct research is not solely a judgment for professionals to make but represents a value judgment which requires the 'informed consent' of society."

As Dr. Katz warms to his subject, the fluidity of his thinking increases, the problems become less esoteric, and the decisions are more urgent. "The basic question gets down to this: what are the permissible limits on experts in our society? In a sense, the medical research community is a state. While we have certain basic safeguards that we wish government states not to transgress in their dealings with their citizens, the professional 'states' are allowed to transgress these safeguards. I'm not satisfied with the argument that the medical profession is doing everything for the best interests and welfare of their patients. The government can say the same thing: we're only doing things for the best interest of our citizens. Over the years we have built up all kinds of safeguards in the law, so why not in the professions? There is today a pernicious climate of excusing all kinds of invasions of people's minds and bodies for the sake of research. This is being done mindlessly and mechanically. It starts in the professional schools where dehumanization is the unspoken basis for professional education. We all must bear some responsibility for changing that."

In the next ten years more research will be needed on

artificial organs, transplants, fetuses, and the unborn—and all can be expected to raise issues regarding their desirability. Innovations must be anticipated now and a plan of action formulated. "Take the atomic bomb, for instance," Dr. Katz observes. "It was developed over a long enough period of time so that position papers should have been written on how we as a society wanted it used, or even if we wanted it used at all. Instead, nothing was done, and Truman had nothing to fall back on. What is needed now are some societal guidelines on experimentation involving genetic defects, artificial organs, methods of behavior control—any one of these may be reality in a very short time."

As complicated as things now are on the human experimentation question, everyone is agreed on at least one thing: things are soon going to get even more complicated as recent technical advances move us closer and closer to the *prediction* of disease, rather than just its diagnosis. New and pernicious forms of experimentation are on the horizon that will pose increasingly subtle and disturbing questions.

The Opening Wedge

At sixty-six years of age James Eslin's grandfather was taken off to a state hospital in the Middle West. During the previous three years he had become forgetful, untidy, incontinent, and given to unpredictable swings in mood. For a long time the doctors hedged on a diagnosis, finally settling on a "form of dementia," a neurologic diagnosis referring to aging and loss of neurons, the brain's specialized nerve cells. Shortly before Mr. Eslin's death, a peculiar twisting motion of his arms and legs developed. At first the motions looked like the nervous fidgeting of a child who finds it difficult to sit at a school desk. But the fidgeting progressed, and finally the old man engaged in a ceaselessly repetitive motion of the arms and legs. Eventually his tongue and face became involved, reducing his already slurred speech to an incomprehensible jumble. Three months later, James Eslin's grandfather was dead.

With James's father, Frank, the onset was different. Fidgeting movements developed when he was about forty-five years old, and co-workers in the life insurance company where Frank was employed noted a strange saluting motion of his right arm. Throughout the day the right arm would move, robotlike, toward his forehead, concluding in a bizarre motion similar to a soldier's salute. Frank, though aware of the motion, was embarrassed and unable to stop it. Within the next few weeks he was seen periodically to furl his eyebrows in deep furrows, as if angry or in pain. This too came and went without purpose or provocation. It was at this time that Frank was asked to speak with the company doctor, who, in turn, requested psychiatric consultation.

On psychiatric examination Frank Eslin didn't fit into any of the standard diagnostic categories. A bit depressed perhaps, but this seemed clearly situational, a response to the "tics" as he called them. Otherwise he was psychiatrically normal. One thing worried the psychiatric consultant, however: Frank seemed to be suffering from the same disease that had killed his father.

Over the next six months, Frank Eslin's erratic movements became more frequent; a new movement appeared, a repetitive shrugging of the shoulders; the facial grimaces and saluting increased in frequency. Eventually Frank Eslin was never free, except when asleep, from one or another of the strange movements.

Shortly before his death Frank was examined by a neurologist, who recognized the movements as symptoms of chorea, a disorder that results from disease in a portion of the brain known as the basal ganglia. In children, chorea can occur in attacks known as Saint Vitus's dance, and it is related to rheumatic fever or infection with a streptococcus bacteria. It is reversible and, with treatment, eventually disappears. But the onset of chorea in adults is usually an ominous sign of serious disease.

Finally, after a conference with the family, Frank was admitted to the hospital for a special neurologic test, a pneumoencephalogram, which involves outlining the brain's inner structures by means of injected air. The test revealed a loss of cells in the special area of basal ganglia known as the caudate nucleus. With these data a diagnosis was possible. Frank and his father before him suffered from Huntington's chorea.

Huntington's chorea is an inherited disease of the nervous system. Symptoms develop in the patient's forties or fifties and progress to mental deterioration and death, usually within ten years. A neurologic textbook describes the patient in the final stages of the disease as "the pitiful picture of the complete ruination of a human being." The patient develops continuous involuntary and uncoordinated movements of the arms, legs, and face, as well as loss of speech and severe mental deterioration ending in insanity. Death by suicide is common, as such patients unfortunately retain until late in the disease a heightened awareness of their own dissolution. Those who do not kill themselves usually die in institutions from infection or from complete exhaustion brought on by the progressing chorea. The two worst features of Huntington's chorea are its hereditary pattern and the absence of a cure.

The inheritance of Huntington's chorea can be traced to families who originally settled in the Boston Bay area and later moved to Suffolk County, New York. There Huntington first described the disease in 1872. (Historical research has uncovered hundreds of victims of the disease who were burned as witches or hanged. One of the best descriptions of the disease can be found in the theological writings of Cotton Mather.)

Inheritance of Huntington's chorea depends on a single gene whose effects are dominant enough to affect roughly half of the family—these are the ones who develop the disease. And herein lies its particularly anguishing nature: no family member can know for certain whether or not he will be likely to develop the feared disease. Each person learns to handle in his own way the dreadful knowledge that a pitiless and incurable process might be stalking him.

James Eslin is now eighteen years old and fully aware that both his grandfather and his father died of Huntington's chorea. But in James's case there is a choice: if he wants to know *now* what fate has in store for him, there is a test that can give him the answer.

In 1970 Dr. Harold Klawans of the University of Chicago formulated a hypothesis about Huntington's chorea. From work with the drug L-Dopa in the treatment of Parkinson's disease, many investigators had reported the onset of a reversible chorea from the use of too much L-Dopa. When the L-Dopa dosage was reduced, the chorea disappeared. L-Dopa seemed to stimulate chorea in susceptible persons. Klawans and his co-workers also knew that L-Dopa increased the chorea in Huntington's chorea. So far, it had never been tried on the relatives at risk for Huntington's chorea. Could L-Dopa be used to detect those who would later develop the disease? Dr. Klawans decided to test his hypothesis.

In 1972 the *New England Journal of Medicine* published Dr. Klawans' study of twenty-eight relatives of patients with known Huntington's chorea. A similar number of normals with no family history of nervous-system disease served as the control group. Each group was placed on a ten-week course of daily L-Dopa; all subjects were checked daily for facial grimaces, tics, and chorea. By the end of the study, 36 per cent of the relatives of Huntington's chorea patients developed one or more signs of the disease. In contrast, none of the healthy controls demonstrated any abnormality. With discontinuance of the test, all signs disappeared.

Thirty-six per cent is uncomfortably similar to the 25 to 50 per cent family incidence of Huntington's chorea. The positive responders, if Dr. Klawans' hypothesis is correct, had briefly experienced some of the signs they would develop in ten or twenty years. Because there is no cure for Huntington's chorea, a positive diagnosis is nothing less than a death sentence.

Tests like Harold Klawans' for the detection of Huntington's chorea are virtually unique. In fact, pretesting for the development of a disease that is still perhaps decades away is something not even imagined ten years ago. In the past, all of us took our chances on what disorders would befall us, and things weren't much more predictable regarding diseases we might later develop than they were about who would die in an automobile accident. Now all that is changing rapidly.

To Marc Lappe of the Hastings Center, pretesting for Huntington's chorea is only "the opening wedge of a movement that will change our ideas of our own humanity." Lappe, an embryologist as well as a bioethicist, sketched for me one snowy day in Hastings, New York, the rough outlines of an impending struggle between our conception of ourselves as self-determining and individualistic and a much darker, grimmer vision where our fates may seem sealed from the moment of our earliest origins: "Data are accumulating to show that certain disease states are not random at all but are correlated with biological markers. There will be more and more cases in the future like Huntington's, where a diagnosis will be made by means of an experimental test ten or maybe even twenty years before the first signs of the disease."

Lappe first came to the Hastings Center in 1971 to take a closer look at the early sickle-cell-testing programs. "I wanted to study this first primordial move to raise people's consciousness that everybody really isn't the same in respect to diseases they may acquire." From his early work at the Institute, Lappe helped draft *Ethical and Social Issues on Screening for Sickle Cell Anemia,* an important but relatively neglected document warning of the abuses of pretesting.

"There is something conceptually very important about having a feeling of autonomy and control over one's destiny and one's body, even one's component parts." Lappe likens much of present-day experimentation to a twentieth-century industrialized society's version of shamanism—the belief among primitive people that possession of any part of a person—a nail, a lock of hair—conveys a power over that person's destiny. "The nail or lock of hair is replaced today by blood samples. From biochemical analysis of blood you can learn things about people that in a very real sense will enable you to maintain some measure of control over them. We're seeing this now in the increasingly sophisticated kinds of data the insurance companies are starting to become interested in. If you turn up with the wrong biochemical data you don't get insurance. Now *that* is having power over people."

As he speaks, Dr. Lappe, who is a youthful, donnish-looking scholar, has a habit of periodically emphasizing his remarks with an exaggerated lift of his eyebrows—a gesture reminiscent of a nun expressing shock or incredulity before an unruly class.

"The possibility of experimenting with people's biologic destiny, telling them *now* what they're likely to develop, even predicting what might kill them—all of this is part of the ancient issue of free will versus determination. Determinism is a looming concept people will not be willing to accept. They are not philosophically ready to deal with a predetermination of their fate.

"Within the last six months, studies on multiple sclerosis, for instance, have shown that it is two different diseases genetically, with two different rates of progression. Certain people are turning out to have an enhanced tendency to develop multiple sclerosis and it takes a more serious form when it does develop. Nor is multiple sclerosis the only disease that may turn out to be strongly predetermined. Certain forms of liver disease are also going the same way. The monamine oxidase content of schizophrenics' blood platelets has recently been found to have possible predictive value, so that one might tell which children of schizophrenics will themselves develop schizophrenia. In all of this, diseases that were believed for centuries to be the result of the environment—something any of us could 'catch'—are turning out to have been inevitable for some people from the beginning. And tests are on the way that will pinpoint who is at risk."

Dr. Lappe paused, arching his eyebrows once more in a final emphatic gesture. "As pretests like the one for Huntington's chorea become available for other diseases, the pressures will build to turn this type of experimentation into practical use. As long as everybody realizes this sort of thing is coming, there may not be any problems. But how many people know about it? And, more importantly, how many of us approve of it? In essence are we philosophically ready for tests pointing to a predetermination of our biological fates? Are we ready to be told *now*, on the basis of an experiment, our biologic destiny? Further, do we have the necessary controls on this new type of experimentation? I think the only candid answer must be no."

Certainly, Lappe's concern about pretesting would establish a much-needed precedent: the anticipation now of ethically complex human experiments that are just in the formative stages. Still, Lappe remains a traditionalist in one important respect: to him experiment chiefly means *medical experiment*, an amalgam of scientists, patients, new drugs, and notebooks of physiologic measurements. But some of the most pernicious studies on human subjects are not medical at all. In addition, they are calling for no less than a redefinition on our part of our concept of "human experiment."

Researchers as Double Agents

In 1970 Laud Humphreys, a sociologist at Southern Illinois University, published in the sociological journal *Trans-Action* the results of a study he had done on homosexuals entitled "Tearoom Trade—Impersonal Sex in Public Places." During the previous two years Humphreys had acted the part of a "watch queen," a homosexual term for a lookout in a rest room who warns of approaching police. "When human behavior is being examined, systematic observation is essential, so I had to become a participant-observer of furtive felonious acts," wrote Humphreys. Apparently he learned his role well, since he observed "hundreds" of homosexual encounters without raising any suspicion regarding his motives. Humphreys' purpose, however, was more involved than just observing and recording patterns of homosexuality. "Although primarily interested in the stigmatized behavior, I also wanted to know about the men who took such risks for a few moments of impersonal sex."

In order to learn more about his subjects, Humphreys noted down their license numbers and, by tracing their cars, learned the identity of his "tearoom" visitors. Then the real experiment began: investigating his subjects' day-to-day lives. For this Humphreys took special precautions. "I changed my hair style, attire, and automobile. I even waited a year between the sample gathering and the interviewing, during which time I took notes of their homes and neighborhoods and acquired data on them from the city and county directories." When this was completed, a disguised Humphreys appeared at his "subjects'" homes for the ostensible purpose of conducting a door-to-door general health survey. Wives, children, and other family members of the subjects were present at the interviews. At no point did Humphreys' questions touch on sexual topics since, in Humphreys' words, "At each level of research I applied those measures which provided maximum protection for research subjects and the truest measurement of persons and behavior observed."

By combining his previous observations in the rest rooms with the newly acquired information on the subjects' everyday lives, Humphreys was able to create a prototype.

Humphreys' experimental method is known as "participant observation," a sociologic experimental method dating from the early 1940s. The key to success in this experimental method is that the distortion resulting from the investigators' being an outside agent is reduced to a minimum. Use of the technique has spread rapidly since its inception, mostly in the social sciences, where it is frequently used. In its barest essentials the method seems harmless enough: care is taken to protect confidentiality; the experimental subjects are not in danger of incurring physical harm; the material gathered in most cases is worthwhile and even unique. But should the concept of "harm" be limited to the infliction of bodily injury?

"Our concept of harm is much too narrow," according to Dr. Katz. "You cannot limit harm in experimental situations to only bodily injury. Even more important are self-determination, privacy, and psychological integrity. This point has not been given the emphasis it deserves. I don't know whether or not I'd call the present explosion of deception experiments unethical, but at least I'd call them abominable."

A shift in emphasis is occurring toward recognizing psychologically "harmful" experimental situations. The most widely publicized experiments embodying potential psychological harm are Stanley Milgram's studies on *Obedience to Authority*. In these, unknowing subjects participated in a phony learning experiment in which the subjects delivered increasing electric shocks under the direction of an experimenter. In actuality the shocks were not real at all, and the person supposedly receiving them was an actor; the experiment was cleverly worked out to test whether or not the volunteers could be made to deliver what they considered were near-fatal electric shocks. Since no real shocks were involved, the point has been made by Milgram and others that the experiments were harmless and worth doing. No measure is included in Milgram's analysis, however, of the psychological harm done to the volunteer subjects, one of whom was told by his wife, "You can call yourself an Eichmann."

To sociologist Kai T. Erikson, such participant observation experiments are "in the very same ethical position as a physician who carries out medical experiments on human subjects without their consent." In "A Comment on Disguised Observation in Sociology," Erikson stated, "It is a matter of cold calculation to point out that this particular research strategy can injure people in ways we can neither anticipate in advance nor compensate for afterward." At the basis of the conflict over participant-observation experiments is the dilemma between individual rights and a scientist's right to know. Humphreys defended his tearoom observations: "Because the majority of arrests on homosexual charges in the United States result from encounters in public rest rooms, I felt this form of sexual behavior to provide a legitimate, even an essential topic for sociological investigation."

For Stanley Milgram his research was not only justified but even contained a moral: "If there is a moral to be learned from the obedience study, it is that every man must be responsible for his own actions. This author accepts full responsibility for the design and execution of the study. Some people may feel it should not have been done. I disagree and accept the burden of their judgment."

But should scientific pursuit of knowledge be allowed to take precedence over the individual's rights to privacy and psychological integrity? What are some of the long-term effects of deception on human experimentation?

An attempt to gauge the subjects' responses to the Milgram experiment was carried out in 1970, when follow-up interviews explored the long-term aftereffects of the experiment. "The most common of them," according to the report, "was the view expressed by approximately half the interviewed subjects that they would now be more suspicious of psychological experiments and more wary about being deceived."

Ironically, the integrity of the experimenters themselves was what had been compromised, the subjects felt. Knowledge was gained at the expense of loss of confidence in scientific research and its methods.

To psychologist Julius Seeman this loss of confidence should not be surprising. He suggests wisdom, not knowledge, as the proper goal of the scientific researcher: "The existence of Hiroshima in man's history demonstrates that knowledge alone is not enough and that the old question of 'knowledge for what?' must still be asked. If knowledge in psychology is won at the cost of some essential humanness in one person's relationship to another, perhaps the price is too high."

The Humphreys and Milgram studies point up the dangers of too narrowly interpreting what constitutes a human subject for experimentation or study. In the past too much emphasis has been on medical research—drugs, hospitals, physicians, and diseases. But human experimentation is not confined to medicine, does not necessarily involve the administration of a drug or chemical, and can even be conducted without any but the most casual contact between experimenter and subject. In a very real sense any one of us, whether at home or at work, in fact in almost any conceivable situation, could be the unknowing participants in "human experimentation." What is worse, no ground rules spell out our rights even in the experiments in which we may *freely* choose to participate. The experimenter may turn out at any time to be a double agent who, under the guise of an "experiment," may seek no less than the exposure of the most fragile and secret recesses of our being.

The Search
for Solutions

While the methods of research and the interests of researchers are changing at a hectic pace, any measures of protection against unethical or even dangerous research have changed little in the twenty years since Irving Ladimer, one of the country's leading legal experts on biomedical research, commented, "There has not yet crystallized a set of specific guidelines commonly understood and applicable to assure that human research may go forward on the highest scientific and ethical planes with due legal protection for both the subject and the investigator." Ladimer's statement is as applicable today as it was in 1954.

The explanation for this inertia can be found, I believe, in an examination of how present research policies have developed. Consider for example the Department of Health, Education, and Welfare's Policy for the Protection of Human Subjects, our primary existing procedural code.

Prior to 1953, the founding of the National Institutes of Health, there were no specific federal or state laws regulating research institutions or investigators using human research subjects. Even more importantly, there seemed to be little interest in drawing up such codes.* In the words of Harvard

---

* In 1960 the NIH sponsored a three-year study by the Boston University Law Medical Research Institution to find out the status of clinical research as actually practiced across the country in the seven years since the founding of the NIH. The Boston study demonstrated conclusively that there was little interest in establishing ethical guidelines in any of

professor William J. Curran, researchers were permitted "to be guided by their own professional judgment and controlled by their own ethical standards as well as those of their institutions." Several converging events were to bring about a change in these attitudes, however.

For one thing, by the early 1960s, the amount of money spent for medical research began to climb astronomically. Over the next ten years the NIH, through its sponsorship of research across the country, was to capture over 50 per cent of the yearly federal budget set aside for research support; the greatest increase was to be in research involving human subjects. Second, organ transplants and more sophisticated surgical techniques demanded policy guidelines as to what would be permissible. In the absence of such guidelines, unfortunate, even ludicrous situations were springing up. For example, the then NIH director, James A. Shannon, was faced in the late 1960s with the problem of a surgeon who had unsuccessfully transplanted an animal kidney into a human recipient "without prior consultation with anybody," in the words of Shannon. Further, "the procedure as performed on the basis of the current information had neither likelihood of therapeutic benefit to the patient nor likelihood of providing new scientific information." In response to incidents like this, the first of many guidelines for human experimentation was drawn up. This sequence of research—abuse of human subjects followed by public outrage followed by guidelines—is a recurring pattern that can be traced from 1953 to the present.

By 1962 the thalidomide scandal had helped bring about the Drug Amendment Act which required the consent of an experimental subject prior to his taking any experimental drug. This brought home the inadequacies of NIH policy regarding informed consent, as well as its continued reliance on the ethical judgment of its individual investigators. No actual change in policy, however, was made until after the occurrence of yet another disastrous research scandal.

In 1963 Drs. Chester M. Southham and Emanuel E.

the eighty-six medical schools queried. All continued to implement NIH policy of placing the primary responsibility for the conduct of research in the hands of the individual investigator.

Mandel were found to have planned and executed a research project at the Jewish Chronic Disease Hospital in Brooklyn, New York (funded by NIH money) in which cancer cells were injected into uninformed subjects. In the wake of great public uproar, both doctors were found guilty of unethical conduct and were censured and placed on probation. Public awareness of the NIH's sponsorship of this research provided the final impetus for the Public Health Service's first official Policy and Procedure Order (PPO 129).

This first research guideline can be summarized briefly as follows: At each facility receiving NIH money an independent "peer review" committee would be set up to assure that "rights and welfare of the subjects would be protected, that the subjects had freely consented to the research, and that the benefits outweighed the risks involved." All subsequent modifications of policy have involved defining and elaborating on these three areas: subject protection, informed consent, and the risk/benefit ratio.

In this first proposal of 1966, for example, it was left to each individual institution to "determine what constitutes the rights and welfare of human subjects in research, what constitutes informed consent, and what constitutes the risks and benefits of a particular investigation." Eight years later in the NIH guidelines of November 1973, our latest federal guidelines on human experimentation, the issue of informed consent was vigorously defined and not left to the vagaries of individual investigator interpretation. "Informed consent has two elements: comprehension of adequate information and autonomy of consent. Consent is a continuing process. The person giving consent must be informed fully of the nature and purpose of the research and of the procedures to be used, including identification of those procedures which are experimental, the possible attendant short- or long-term risks and discomforts, the anticipated benefits to himself and/or others, any alternative methods of treatment, expected duration of the study, and of his or her freedom to ask any questions and to withdraw at any time, should the person wish to do so. There must also be written evidence of the process used for obtaining informed consent, including grounds for belief that the subject has understood the information given, and has sufficient maturity and mental capacity to make such choices and formulate the requisite judgment to consent. In addition, the person must have sufficient autonomy to choose, without duress, whether or not to participate."

In the years since the first HEW policy statement, interest in the regulation of human experimentation has become worldwide. In 1964 the World Medical Association issued the Declaration of Helsinki, which permitted experiments "with the subjects' consent and if the experiment could be justified on therapeutic grounds." That same year, the Medical Research Council in England stated that "the true consent of the subject must be explicitly obtained." In those cases where the patient could not be expected to benefit personally from the research, the requirement was even more vigorous: "If he is to submit to it he must volunteer in the full sense of the word." Other professional groups soon followed with their own contributions to regulating human experimentation—in all, thirty-eight proposals.

Throughout these various proposals several simple basic principles reappear. For one thing, the research subject must be a volunteer who has been given all the information necessary to make an informed decision; he should be free to withdraw from participation at any point in the experiment which has been so designed to have eliminated through prior animal experiments all unnecessary risk; the benefits of the experiment should outweigh the risk to the experimental subject; and the experiment should be conducted by qualified scientists.

With such unanimity in principle among the various proposals, one would think it possible to draw up a final, all-encompassing regulation for human experimentation. So far, this has been impossible for several reasons. For one thing, the definition of a "volunteer" is not nearly as easy to come up with as it first appears. Can a prisoner or mental patient be a "volunteer"? The Detroit psychosurgery case and the U.S. Bureau of Prisons' Project START suggest that people living within an "inherently coercive" atmosphere cannot be "volunteers" in any meaningful sense of the word.

THE ANIMAL OF NECESSITY

Can children give free consent to be volunteers? If not, do their parents have the right to volunteer them for an experiment? Finally, the suggestion that the benefits of an experiment can supersede the risks to the individual subject is thought by many to be inconsistent with the principle of inalienable rights.

Applying some of these criticisms to the Tuskegee syphilis study highlights the general vagueness and uselessness of these guidelines. If informed consent was to have any meaning, how could impoverished and uneducated blacks from rural Alabama be selected in the first place? How could the risks inherent to the participant in Tuskegee have been weighed against the expected advancement in medical knowledge? In any event, how are "risks," "benefits," and the "importance of knowledge" to be evaluated and weighed one against the other? In fact, can the possibility of harm to a research subject ever be outweighed by the gaining of knowledge, however important scientifically?

In response to such criticisms, HEW has been working for the past year on a new guideline for human experimentation. The result is the Protection of Human Subjects, Policies and Procedures. According to these guidelines, revised on May 30, 1974, the safeguards of the rights of experimental subjects "will be the organization which receives or is accountable to HEW." In order to facilitate this, funds from HEW would be refused to any research organization which has not "reviewed and approved" the proposed activities. This will be done principally by ethical committees composed of both professional and nonprofessional members. Specifically excluded under the new proposal are committees composed entirely of research personnel. "No committee shall consist entirely of a single professional group," according to the proposal. It will be the review committee's job to keep HEW informed of problems via periodic review of ongoing research. This will "ascertain the acceptability of proposals in terms of organizational commitments and regulations, applicable laws, standards of professional conduct and practice, and community attitudes." For the first time, protections are included for children, prisoners, the institutionalized, the fetus, and the products of abortion.

Several criticisms have been leveled at the new policy. First, its restriction to HEW-funded research greatly limits its usefulness as a potential regulator of research done by other government agencies, such as the Bureau of Prisons and LEAA. Second, the placement of responsibility for research formulation on the recipients of HEW grants may lead to each institution's setting up its own ethical standards. Critics suggest that only a centralized ethical standard board would be satisfactory. Third, there are no enforcement provisions that would eliminate the possibility of unethical experiments being conducted with HEW funds. Finally, some feel that where protection of human subjects is concerned, there is no place for balancing "the importance of knowledge to be gained" against risks to the individual subject.

I discussed the latest HEW Policies and Procedures for the Protection of Human Subjects guidelines with Donald Chalkley, chief of the Institutional Relations Branch of the National Institutes of Health. A tall middle-aged man with a deep sonorous voice and thick wavy hair, Dr. Chalkley can summon up on command a total recall of cases involving human experimentation, his field of specialization since 1956.

According to Dr. Chalkley, some of the most fundamental issues at stake in human experimentation are always going to be clouded by ambiguity and confusion. Even something as simple as deciding on what constitutes the "community" where the experiment will be carried out can be tricky and fraught with conflict. "Take Johns Hopkins Hospital, for instance," he says. "Here is one of the largest hospitals in the world dedicated to human experimentation. It is demanded under the new proposal that research conducted at Hopkins should reflect the value systems of the local community. But determining the people who make up that 'community' involves several inherent contradictions. Because Johns Hopkins is a medical mecca it attracts people irrespective of geography—they come from every country in the world for inpatient treatment. But Hopkins' outpatient population is restricted to a small part of Baltimore, Maryland. Now what 'community' are we referring to when we speak of the needs or the wishes on human experimentation of the 'community' of Johns Hopkins Hospital? We hear a lot these days about the hospital conforming to its 'community.' Now I ask you, what *community*?"

Dr. Chalkley cites the experience of Dr. Joseph Goldzieher as another example of the problems that can arise between a hospital and the "community." In 1972 Dr. Goldzieher set up a study in Texas to evaluate whether the side effects of "the pill" were physical or psychological. Mexican-American women workers were divided into two groups, the first receiving the birth-control pill, the second a placebo. (Both groups were told to use vaginal foams since the pills might not be "completely effective.") In response to criticism by the Population Council of the casual oral-consent procedure that was used with the women, a written protocol and consent form were developed. This was translated at the University of Texas into Castilian Spanish and given to the women, all of whom of course spoke that mixture of Mexican, Spanish, and English known as "Tex Mex." Ironically, the patients were better equipped to read English than Castilian Spanish, a fact eventually pointed out by a businessman serving on the hospital committee. "This is a clear-cut demonstration that the researchers were living in an ivory tower," Dr. Chalkley observed. "The Spanish department of the university, as well as the hospital, didn't even know what kind of Spanish was spoken by the local citizens! For all practical purposes the hospital and the community were light-years apart."

The diversity of communities in different parts of the country also makes rigid membership requirements unrealistic, says Dr. Chalkley. "Let's assume for a moment you want to set up a committee to evaluate a research proposal and that you want representatives on that committee of both women and blacks. What would be more natural than to choose a black woman lawyer, for instance? But let's face it, in many institutions in the Deep South it isn't that easy to find a black woman lawyer. If such a person is a requirement for a local committee, then she will have to be brought in from somewhere else. But in what sense will such 'circuit riders' represent the local community?"

Dr. Chalkley is also uncomfortable with what he sees as an overdependence on legal sanctions, since the law is conservative and traditional. "One thing disturbs me about passing laws about human experimentation: the law is built to deal with phenomena after they have occurred. While we are moving toward preventive medicine, very little is being done about a preventive-medical law. Reliance is still placed on the threat of consequences if something goes wrong. Penalties are there after the fact. I would like to see the emphasis on intelligent steps to insure that bad effects do not occur, rather than the present preoccupation with the issue of who is at fault when something goes wrong."

Certainly the history of laws applying to medicine is filled with embarrassing examples of the law lagging behind medical progress. Preschool vaccination for smallpox still remains a requirement in many states, despite recommendations by the Public Health Service that smallpox vaccination be omitted, even for foreign travelers: at risk is a small but significant number who will develop a severely disabling and often fatal encephalitis as a result of the vaccination. In California an outdated law forbids the administration of more than 80 per cent oxygen to premature infants, despite demonstrations that the respiratory distress syndrome of infancy responds best to a brief exposure to 90 per cent oxygen. "These cases illustrate the truth behind the old legal adage that it's easy to pass a bad law but it's difficult to get a bad law off the books," Dr. Chalkley noted in exasperation.

Another area of legal overemphasis is the issue of informed consent. "We're hearing a lot now about informed consent and, of course, it is important. But any doctor will tell you, if he's frank, that obtaining consent is not that much of a problem, no matter what research is proposed. We've seen this with researchers who never fail to obtain valid consent from their patients, even after consultants advised them strongly against participating in the experiment. We must remember that some people have a tendency to regard research doctors almost like gods and are willing to consent to whatever they think the researcher wants." A more important issue, according to Dr. Chalkley, is the weighing of risks against the possible benefit to the patient, the so-called risk-benefit ratio. "The problem is really not with the integrity of the medical profession in seeking the consent, but with whether or not they really know all of the problems before they undertake research. My concern is with the ignorance inevitable and inherent in research."

All previous attempts to regulate human research originate from this concern to balance the gains from the research against the risks involved. One response in the past has been to deny and ignore the risks. As a result we have had Tuskegee, with bad results. Now some are urging that the responsibility for research be taken out of the hands of the scientific community altogether. But Dr. Chalkley thinks this is an overreaction, throwing out the baby with the bath water. "The strongest contribution of the scientific community comes from the in-depth exploration that a group of specialized scholars can do with a research proposal. They can do a much better job than any group of nonscientists. A council of laymen replacing a study section of biomedical scholars will deprive the public of about fifty per cent of the protection it has already. Consider a typical experiment. Ninety babies—all potential victims of constrictive pericarditis, which can end in sudden death. You know from experience that only a third of them will have the disease. You, as the researcher, propose to determine whether or not a biopsy can diagnose the condition. This carries a one-half of one per cent mortality risk, but you can save eighty per cent of the lives at risk. You are faced with a very practical decision—whether the risk to two-thirds justifies the benefit to the other third of the babies. I don't see how anyone without an in-depth knowledge of the procedures involved is going to come up with the risk-benefit figures which may precede any consideration of informed consent. In this case—an actual proposed experiment—it was decided that the risks were too high and the thing never got as far as determining informed consent."

Whatever the mechanisms of protection offered, can a set of absolute rules for human experimentation be achieved? At this point nobody knows. Two different legal proposals have been in the forefront of consideration recently.

The first, the Protection of Human Subjects Act, H.R.7724, sponsored by Senator Edward Kennedy, was passed by both the House and Senate and signed into law on July 12, 1974. It establishes an eleven-member commission chosen from the general public and from individuals in specified fields such as medicine, law, ethics, and theology. The committee's initial task will be "to undertake a comprehensive investigation and study to develop the basic ethical principles which should underlie the conduct of biomedical and behavioral research involving human subjects and develop and implement policies and regulations to insure that such research is carried out in accordance with the ethical principles established by the commission." Included in the commission's responsibilities are setting up a comprehensive study to pinpoint the ethical principles underlying clinical research; appointing institutional review boards within all research institutions; defining more precisely the interface between biomedical and behavior research and the everyday practice of medicine.

A unique feature of the Kennedy bill is a "mechanism for the compensation of individuals and their families for injuries . . . or death caused by participating . . . in a biomedical or behavioral research program." No previous guideline has provided financial assistance for those injured during experimental procedures.

Patients' rights are protected under the Kennedy bill by a Subject Advisory Committee "primarily concerned with the protection of the rights of subjects of biomedical and behavioral research." It would function independently of the research investigators and would try to provide potential subjects with "total disclosure" of the risks they ran.

Although we should be grateful for the Kennedy bill as a start toward the regulation of human experimentation, it has several major weaknesses. For one thing it is limited to health-science programs funded in whole or in part by the Department of Health, Education, and Welfare. Compliance with the bill cannot be demanded of privately funded research groups or even of research conducted within other branches of the government. Now many behavior-modification experiments are taking place under the sponsorship of the Bureau of Prisons, but the Kennedy bill would not regulate abuses in that area. So far, no legislation has been introduced by anyone that would regulate human experimentation at all times and under all circumstances.

Second, the commission's authority is poorly defined, carrying no real power to enforce compliance. If experimenters chose to ignore the commission and its recommendations, not much could be done about it. Also, the bill contains no provision for publication and dissemination of the commission's decisions, which would be essential to drawing up national guidelines that could be applied by all researchers. Finally, and to many critics, most importantly, the bill depends upon the "good faith" of biotechnical researchers. Dr. Barber's studies, as well as the pathetic history of human experimentation, cast serious doubt on the advisability of basing a regulatory bill on anybody's "good faith."

The second regulatory proposal is largely the work of Dr. Jay Katz of Yale and Professor Alexander Capron of the University of Pennsylvania Law School. Capron, a former law student of Katz's at Yale in the late 1960s, has continued to collaborate with his old mentor on the subject of their shared concern: human experimentation. Together they have come up with a proposal calling for a National Human Investigation Board composed of "eminent medical and other professional researchers and lay members who can represent the interests of society or the ethical conduct of research with human subjects." Dividing all research projects into formulation, administration, and review, the NHIB would restrict nonmedical participation to the areas of formulation and review in which nonscientists have most to contribute. Administration would be performed by the researcher's professional peers sitting on institutional review committees.

The tasks of the proposed NHIB would include: the selection of subjects, with an emphasis on "reexamining the contemporary research practice of choosing subjects from the less educated, disadvantaged or captive groups with society"; reformulating "informed consent," with special emphasis on "the nature and quality of the interactions between investigator and subject"; a clarification between "research" activities and the more routine, medically accepted procedures (in the past, blurring the distinction between "treatment" and "research" has enabled some investigators to carry out experimental studies without previously submitting a research protocol) ; and drawing up acceptable risk-benefit criteria. The Board would try to answer such questions as: What is an acceptable risk? How often can risky experiments be repeated to duplicate already known results? What rules will apply to healthy subjects engaged in a research project? Will higher risks be allowable with patient subjects who might stand to gain directly from the research? The Board would also establish "no fault" clinical research insurance which would be paid for by the institution conducting the research and provide full protection for subjects as well as eliminating the need to prove negligence or malpractice in the event of a research injury; and it would promulgate sanctions for noncompliance with research standards. These might be simply peer review or, more seriously, discontinuance of federal or private research funding, or, in some cases, even criminal prosecution.

The actual administration of NHIB would involve Institutional Human Investigation Committees (IHIC) to replace the present unspecialized institution-review committees. The IHIC would be responsible for the general conduct of research in any institution, and policies would be reviewed and approved by the Board.

At the level where the specialized formulation of research protocols takes place, a Protocol Review Group (composed entirely of scientists and experts) would provide the scientific knowledge necessary to arrive at decisions such as risk-benefit ratios. Procedures are also proposed for investigator education on responsible human research, mechanisms of appeal (even a "supreme court"), and publication of research decisions.

So far, the National Human Investigation Board has not developed beyond the talking stage. What makes it of compelling interest is everyone's conviction that something must be done about human experimentation. But what? And when?

To Alexander Capron, the ultimate solution to the human experimentation question may be further off in the future than any of us realize. But he has launched an outspoken campaign for the establishment of the National Human Investigation Board. Despite his youth—he is a tall, gangly blond with a striking resemblance to Van Cliburn—Capron commands respect here and in Europe for the vigor of his proposals. While many are indecisively floundering around, Capron is steadily coming closer to workable solutions.

"I like to think of the work of the NHIB as medically rivaling in importance the work of the Supreme Court. Traditionally the Supreme Court does not pass on issues that turn exclusively on factual data of guilt or culpability. Rather it concerns itself with the questions of broad legal importance. I think that the National Human Investigation Board should function like the Supreme Court by evaluating the major policy issues surrounding human experimentation."

Capron's proposed "supreme court" can be illustrated by a research proposal he encountered at a neighboring university medical center. "A very reputable scientist was proposing a study of the effects of a seventy-two-hour starvation diet on the fetuses of a group of women about to undergo elective abortions. The protocol called for the admission of the women to the hospital, their volunteering and participating in the seventy-two-hour starvation, followed by a tissue examination on the aborted fetus.

"Now a protocol like that may be considered perfectly ethical in one research center, while another may object, for instance, that the women had no right to impose such an experiment on the fetus. Scientists in a third research center may say, 'The fetus is going to be aborted anyway, so what does it matter?' I think a National Human Investigation Board would be able to take a research problem like that and come up with a policy decision that could then become universal."

Turning his attention to experiments in children, his special area of expertise, Capron has even come up with a set of guidelines regulating pediatric drug studies. "Today parents are given astounding powers of control over their children. Legally it is an unsettled question as to whether or not this is proper. There are no safeguards now to rule out instances in which the parents' decision stems from a desire to punish or hurt the child, or with other pathological intents. Admittedly, these instances are rare, but we need a framework for rare occurrences as well as for the everyday."

Capron wants methods that will "randomize" the children selected for research. "There are many situations in society where membership in a group implies obligations in return for sharing in the benefits conferred by membership. The military draft is a good example. I'm thinking of a method of randomly selecting children for inclusion in experimentation. So far, frankly, I haven't come up with any that would stand up under legal challenge."

Capron is not alone in being unable to devise guidelines that will work at all times and under all circumstances. The very concept of human experimentation—subjecting people to treatments and investigative studies whose final results must remain speculative—precludes the drawing up of facile panaceas. Its importance, however, lends a note of urgency to all ongoing attempts to establish the guidelines. Whether by means of the Kennedy bill or the Katz-Capron Human Investigation Board, control must one day be achieved.

"Admittedly, the answers are hard to come up with," reflects Dr. Katz. "But that shouldn't keep us from striving for guidelines to safeguard the three interests at stake in any human experimentation—the subject, the investigator, and most importantly, all the rest of us. For we now must formulate the attitudes and guidelines that will serve as the final determinants of what one man will be able to do to another in the name of experimentation."

Within the last two years a radically different solution has been proposed for the problems raised by human experimentation and biomedical technology.

In 1971 Paul Sieghart, a London lawyer, organized a group composed of three scientists, two moral philosophers, a psychiatrist, and a lawyer. "What we were after was a practical means for the performance of the social obligations of scientists."

First, Sieghart and his "working party," as he termed

THE ANIMAL OF NECESSITY

it, took up the issue of whether or not scientists have a special obligation in terms of the consequences of their work. In the past, many scientists have argued that their responsibility stops with the development of a scientific breakthrough. What use is made of that breakthrough, they claim, is irrelevant to their aims. To Sieghart, this argument was less than appealing. "A good starting point for deciding whether anyone has a special moral obligation to others is to ask whether he is especially well placed to benefit or harm them." According to Sieghart, laws regulating such things as speed limits on highways and the professional relations of a doctor with his patient rest largely on the harmful consequences that can result from carelessness. Scientific work must be included in such a scheme. "The outcome of scientific work can often have a great impact for good or ill on other people. Quite frequently scientists can predict this outcome earlier and more accurately than others. Sometimes they can even modify the results. One could claim, therefore, that scientists are in one of the special positions which give rise to special obligations."

As a starting point, Sieghart's "working party" listed several special obligations of scientists to society.

First, a scientist could refuse to engage in certain lines of scientific investigation. Although much scientific work, particularly basic scientific investigation, does not have immediate social application, other research is socially relevant, such as research on nerve gases or weaponry. In these situations, Sieghart held, the scientist considers the option of refusing to participate. "Such a gesture can be socially important because it helps to improve the moral climate so that it comes to seem less respectable for scientists to do that kind of work."

Closely allied with refusal to engage in socially pernicious research is the second obligation: to influence other scientists to think out the consequences of planned research. "We believe that anyone who engages in activity which might have harmful social consequences ought to apply his mind to those consequences and to act on his conclusions. We do not think it is good enough to put on blinders, concentrating on the job in hand and leaving the consequences to others."

Finally, the scientist must make active efforts to in-form the public of the likely consequences of new biotechnological developments. "Society should have the opportunity as soon as possible to reinforce the research effort and to prepare the means for utilizing the benefits and making them available to its members. . . . Society must have time to work out an intelligent response in advance by initiating whatever research is necessary to get as clear an idea of what the consequences are likely to be, and what needs to be done about them."

By Sieghart's own admission, his list of "special obligations" was at first pretty much a trial balloon, an intellectual exercise in an area that interested him. But Sieghart found himself increasingly caught up with the urgency of the problem. After reviewing the situation in London, for instance, he found little or no communication between scientists and his own colleagues engaged in law and the ongoing machinery of government. In a word, the situation was chaotic. In addition, the scientists interested in the social application of their research had no organized means of bringing this to public attention.

"Scientific work which may have a great impact on all our lives is being done all over the world. The scientists who are doing this work may well be aware of the possible dangers. But at the moment there is little the individual scientist can do in this respect between the extremities of a sensational newspaper article and a discreet letter to a member of parliament."

Even when the issues are clear-cut (certainly a rare situation in bioethics), biomedical catastrophes often prove almost irreversible. "It is not until the potential dangers become apparent through some scandal or disaster that they catch the attention of the popular press and there is a public outcry. At that point it is often too late. Too many people or organizations have acquired a vested interest in the discovery or its development to make it possible to deprive them of its fruits." Examples of the type of situation mentioned by Sieghart include the early contraceptive pills, with their alarming incidence of vascular complications, or the burgeoning field of computer data banking which is only now receiving the scrutiny it deserves as a major threat to individual privacy and autonomy. In each of these instances, vested interest groups, after putting in money and effort, can be counted on to provide stern opposition to any challenges. The key element here, according to Sieghart, is *early* intervention. "We need to intervene at a time when the process has not yet gathered enough momentum to be beyond our control."

All of this eventually led Paul Sieghart to make a unique proposal for the control of biomedical technology. In the September 1972 issue of *Nature,* Sieghart proposed setting up a new institution with the task of "stimulating informed public discussion about the possible consequences of socially important pieces of scientific research, in each case at its earliest possible moment." (In the early draft the institution is called Science and Society Council; it was later changed to the Council for Science and Society.) Although it has been in operation for less than a year, it is the most exciting and promising venture yet toward humanizing biomedical technology.

The secretary of the new council is Jerome K. Ravetz, a transplanted Philadelphian who came to England as a Fulbright scholar in the McCarthy days and has stayed ever since. The author of *Scientific Knowledge and Its Social Problems,* Ravetz is considered by many to be "radical" or at the very least "non-establishment" in his allegiances, which have in the past included the British Society for Social Responsibility in Science (BSSRS), an early effort directed toward similar ends, but also including dramatic and highly controversial examples of political activism.

During my research for this book I spent several days with Ravetz, a puckish, bearded man in his early forties. Involvement with the council has cost Ravetz friends; many say he has "sold out" by agreeing to participate on a council which includes such an establishment figure as its chairman, the president of the BBC, Sir Michael Swan.

"I look upon my own predicament as similar to the criticism that was leveled at the American clergy in the early sixties," says Ravetz. "Many people were critical of them for getting involved with social issues, urging instead they stick to their churches. Now we realize that religion has to be involved with social issues. So too must science. The innocent happy days of pure science are over. In a sense, scientists are political animals, influenced by social trends and, in turn, bringing a great influence to bear on society."

Ravetz's own reason for joining the council include recognition that change has to be brought about *within* the system. It implies, therefore, a willingness to meet and exchange ideas with those wielding power within the system.

The essence of the council's work will be the anticipation of the social effects of biomedical technology. In order to do this, scientists will be invited, in fact many volunteer on their own, to present drafts on research in progress. They will be scholarly, technical, and have little reference to social applications. Other experts may then be called in to contribute a "state of the art" document. Then the real work of the council will begin. "You must remember," insists Ravetz, "we're eventually aiming at a transformation of highly technical concepts into something that can be read and understood by someone reading between tube stations. The 'working party' assigned this formidable task of translation will not be 'experts' but a group of intelligent people with different backgrounds, swapping their insights on the problems presented by the scientists. Their proposals will be kicked around, discussed, refined, speculated on, until eventually we've achieved a mature, broad-based analysis." The council's opinion will be published (including minority opinions, which in some cases may go so far as a disclaimer), and after that, Ravetz hopes, the council's work will stimulate public opinion via television and the press. "At this point the issues will not be so much scientific as political. What do the people *really* think about test-tube babies, for instance? Right now the average person doesn't even have an opinion, because he thinks of it as something out of science fiction instead of an area of active research that demands immediate attention."

If the council's work is successful, Ravetz foresees a shifting of responsibility from scientists themselves to the public at large. "Now, the only responsibility is responsibility to the paymaster. Scientists have to devise research protocols that will obtain funding. Beyond that there is no responsibility. Do you know what the paradigm of power without responsibility is?" Ravetz asks impishly. "It's the prostitute: great power without a corresponding responsibility. So far, science has functioned like a prostitute."

While the drawing up of laws and guidelines seems to be the order of the day in the United States, the British emphasis is against legal constraints. Ravetz does not envision the council's lobbying for the passage of regulatory bills. "You must remember, professional reputation is extremely important in the scientific community. All that is really needed to stop certain lines of research is to create a general odor of distaste. There are subtle and not so subtle ways of saying, 'Look, here is a line of research we don't want pushed; there are other areas deserving of more effort.' In essence, you get the idea around that certain areas of research are under suspicion, as with heart transplants, which are not currently scientifically respectable. No laws were passed, in fact a surgeon is free to do one today if he wishes, but the general climate is so unfavorable to such an operation that for all practical purposes heart transplants have ceased."*

For another example of the effectiveness of the method, Ravetz points to the work of his colleague on the council, Sir Michael Swan. As leader of a government inquiry in 1972 into the use of antibiotics in animal foodstuffs, Swan spearheaded a successful effort to restrict antibiotic-"spiked" grains.

How would the council actually work? A typical example, Paul Sieghart suggests, is the issue of parents' predetermination of the sex of their children. As a first step, scientists engaged in research in this area would be asked to present position papers to a working party of the council—composed in this case of, say, a gynecologist, a psychiatrist, a sociologist, and a lawyer. Next, a small but adequate sociologic survey would be conducted to find out how people feel about such a technique, whether they would use it, and what sex child

---

* Ravetz was proved correct within a month of this statement when a heart transplant, Britain's first in three years, ended in the death of the recipient. Television commentators as well as the editorial staff of *The Times* of London publicly raised the question of the propriety of this operation.

they might select. Suppose, Sieghart suggests, that the survey turned out to indicate that twice as many parents would choose boys over girls. Two courses of action would then be possible: either let the sex predetermination go forward, or suggest methods of stopping it (presupposing other surveys indicating an unfavorable overall effect from having twice as many men as women). "Since the matter of sex predetermination is one of major public interest, the press and other media can be relied on to give it ample publicity. From that point on, the normal democratic process can take over. The matter will become one of continuing discussion in the press and in the departments of government most concerned. By the processes with which we are all familiar, the response thought to be most apt for our particular society can evolve, and eventually any necessary legislation can be passed."

After six months of intensive study and "brain picking" among Britain's scientific establishment, Ravetz and Sieghart have focused on six issues that demand the council's immediate attention. "As you can see, we've omitted things like cloning, which might be key issues for the council in ten years. We can't afford the luxury of speculating that far ahead now. Too many things need immediate answers." The six issues are: the standards to be applied and procedures for applying them in weighing "acceptable risk" from pollution against anticipated benefits from new technologies; the use of surgical, pharmacological, psychological, and other techniques for the control of individual behavior deemed to be harmful or deviant; the contradictions implicit in the search for "harmless" weapons for the control of civil disorder; the problem posed to successful communication by the rapid growth in the volume of published technical information; the social and ethical implications of the nonclinical use of mood-control drugs; and the problem of monitoring technologies in instances where technical competence is monopolized by a small number of institutions committed to the same interest.

The proposals of the council in their final form would include the social consequences of a particular line of research. In addition, council recommendations would include measures that could be taken if predicted social consequences were thought to be undesirable. Finally, the probable consequences of any preventive measures would also be spelled out. Sieghart says: "The important point for our purpose is that, as a result of our work, the public debate and the political decision-making process will be based on a better knowledge of the relevant facts, will begin much earlier, and will have more chance to lead to a policy that is properly thought out."

Although the council is a tremendous step forward in gaining public participation, some think it is still too narrowly based to be effective. Typical of this view is that of Steven Rose, co-founder of the BSSRS. Although a powerful intellectual figure within the London scientific community, Rose has not been asked to join the council, perhaps in tacit recognition of his publicly expressed criticism of its chances for success. In the last five years Rose, a thirty-five-year-old biochemist and brain scientist who recently wrote a book entitled *The Conscious Brain,* has devoted much of his time to collaborative efforts with his wife, Hilary, a sociologist. Together they wrote *Science and Society,* which contains many ideas similar to those adopted by the council. Tall, athletically built, Rose can be a formidable figure in debate, concealing as he does a stunning intelligence behind the trappings of a rather brash insouciance. At times Rose can be impatient, supercilious, and downright overbearing. Not surprisingly, this has not endeared him to many members of the council.

Two days after speaking with Ravetz, I spent an afternoon with Steven Rose, who outlined his objections to the council: "The council is bound to be ineffectual because it includes members who are irrevocably committed to shoddy science and to avoiding key issues. For instance, one of the members of the council is the director of one of the largest environmental pollutants in all of Britain. In addition, the council implies a ready acceptance of the view that society is a given, that society as presently structured is fine and science should be brought into conformity with it. I think that particular assumption is the most objectionable of all. The questions we have to ask in the long run are: what sort of science do we want? How much of it do we want? Who should do it? How should they and their activities be controlled? But the most fundamental question underlying all of this is: what sort of *society* do we want?"

In his books and published statements Rose has called attention to one of our most cherished and enduring myths: the neutrality of science. All of us have tucked away in the back of our minds the image of a scientist working away in isolation toward the discovery of "truth." What directions his research may take; what scientific "truths" he may arrive at; what research questions he may ask—somehow all these matters seem predetermined by the "scientific method," far removed, for instance, from social and political processes. But this is of course not true. As Rose puts it, "In fact, the problems we have now do not derive from some mad scientist closeted in a lab and doing research that is particularly dangerous. The problem is that specific decisions are being made every day, capriciously, even irresponsibly, toward supporting research in particular directions."

As Rose points out, there are historical precedents for a socially derived science. Because the ancient Babylonians believed in the possibility of predicting heavenly events, they poured huge sums of money into astronomy. With the industrial revolution in the nineteenth century, advanced power generation became necessary, which led to research being done on the laws of thermodynamics and the conservation of energy. "The question should be whether the sort of society we want should shape our choice of technologies, or whether we should allow our society to be shaped by the 'inevitability' of technological advance."

Looked at from Rose's perspective, the emphasis of the council is all wrong. In his opinion, the working parties should be set up around the issues of desired social change, with biomedical technology only providing the "hardware" necessary to bring those changes about. "The question of biomedical technology is not so much a question of knowledge as it is of control. What controls exist now are in the hands of the powerful members of society. This leaves us with two problems: how to democratize knowledge and how to democratize these controls."

The individual scientist, according to Rose, must bear the brunt of democratizing knowledge. He should not be involved in "secret" research; he should not accept funding from sources that oppose the interests of democratization of science. "In summary, he must see to it that his specialized knowledge is as widely and publicly disseminated as possible." Naturally such democratization of knowledge will involve scientists in a new relationship with the public. In a sense they will become advocates, pushing for certain lines of research, engaging in pressure groups, eventually even agitation. To Rose this change in orientation is imminent, challenging, and highly desirable. "Science is one special-interest group among many. In fact, more money for science, or for anything else, is the cry of an interest group."

Most interest groups, when recognized for what they are, must provide justification for their continued support. Science looked upon as "neutral" and "inevitable" has long been exempt from public accountability. Only after the thalidomide disaster, for instance, were we made aware of the tremendous lack of controls on the marketing of drugs. By now the pattern has become predictable: decisions are made by scientists with no contribution from the public; they are followed by a disaster, public alarm, and the setting of "watchdog" institutions. Now Rose and others are suggesting a fundamental change in the pattern: let the public in on the decision from the beginning. "It is this inaccessibility which lies at the root of the problem of contemporary science and its social relations. At a time of rapid technological change, in which the world is being continuously reshaped around us and not always for the better, the key processes of this reshaping are inaccessible."

Although deeply divided on methods, both the members of the council and Steven Rose are united in their aim for greater public participation in scientific decision making. In Rose's words, "Mechanisms have to be found for identifying potential technological developments and for public assessment of their desirability and priority."

Devising the means to achieve these goals has only just started. The work could not be more important. "That man and his planet survive is a continuing tribute to luck, human ingenuity, and society's adaptive capacity," says Rose. "We cannot rely on the permanent success of this combination."

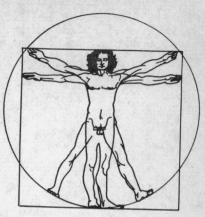

The
Only <u>Real</u>
Solution

In the two years I spent researching and writing this book, my own thinking has undergone considerable revision. I started out with the rather naive assumption that scientific expertise coupled with a reasonable amount of goodwill could go a long way toward solving the problems of biomedical technology. If we have been able to overcome the enormously difficult obstacles in developing technologies of genetic modification and prediction, behavior control, and new tools of experimentation, then, I reasoned, the issue of defining limits and goals would be easy in comparison. This was indeed a gratuitous and illogical assumption. I am no longer confident that the problems of controlling biomedical technology will take care of themselves. In fact, the immediate future may portend fewer rather than more controls.

The list of potential horrors—*in vitro* fertilization, anonymous sperm banking, behavior-control technology in the prisons and ghettos, experiments on unwitting human subjects—is lengthening, and yet we are as far as ever from unified policies. More importantly, there seems to be no hope in the near future for a workable solution to the problems presented by these biomedical technologies. Where are we going? Who is in charge? There are no answers to these questions.

In the last two years, thanks to astute public-service journalism, many abuses have been brought to public attention and halted temporarily. Psychosurgery in prisons, for example, has not been carried out in the last year, at least so far as I can determine. No established guidelines exist, however, to insure its permanent abandonment. So, too, with experimentation with the mentally retarded.

At this point I don't propose to trot out a ten- or twenty-point program that will solve all the problems mentioned in this book. I wish I could do that. But, in fact, I don't believe there are any absolute answers, at least I haven't found them after interviewing several hundred scientists and others who have thought about these problems. Moreover, some of the problems are harder to solve than others. In behavior control and genetic engineering, for instance, certain courses of action seemed reasonable to me; these have already been given in Parts one and two of this book. Things are a lot more difficult, however, with human experimentation. Controls in this area are going to be incredibly complicated, given our present need for newer and more effective treatments for crippling fatal diseases.

In the case of children, for example, the dilemma may be insoluble because meaningful drug research intended to benefit children can often be carried out only with children as research subjects. (Doses, response patterns, side effects, and idiosyncratic reactions all differ in children as compared to adults.) Along with our awareness of the child's unique metabolic response has come a corresponding awareness of the child's right not to be experimented upon. Proxy consent is proving invalid and soon parental consent will not be acceptable as a justification for a child's participation in experiments. All of this may lead to a ticklish situation indeed: the prohibition of research on children might spell the end of twenty years of ongoing study directed to the cure of leukemia, for example. On the other hand, to allow research on children implies, at least implicitly, a willingness to sacrifice the autonomy if not the lives of certain children in order to achieve a cure for childhood leukemia. But whose children?

A closely related area is the search for a cure for other forms of cancer. We all agree on the importance of finding a cure for the nation's number-two killer. But by what ground rules will this cure be achieved? Do we want it badly enough to sanction any experiment, however dangerous, however it may disregard human rights? If we do, then the ongoing attempts to control and regulate human experimentation can rightfully be regarded as obstructionist. But if the cure for cancer is not desirable "at any price," then experimental guidelines should now be formulated to set limits on what is and what is not allowable.

After considerable thought and debate, I have become convinced that the British Council for Science and Society, although not perfect, is currently the best approach we have for gaining control over biomedical technology. Sieghart and Ravetz have grasped the essential point: the control and regulation of biomedical technology must ultimately rest with nonscientists and "non-experts." Through polls, action groups, or perhaps even a national referendum, the wishes of the majority must be sampled. In the United States such efforts have already culminated in a Supreme Court decision on the issue of abortion. Similar public advocacy, debate, even political agitation, is called for on other biomedical questions. In essence we must develop a correlate for biomedical technology of a civil rights act that will free us all from the potential oppression that can be visited on us by a biomedical technology out of control. For some, it is almost too late. In the case of our brothers in prison, for instance, or those brought low by grinding poverty, biomedical technology is already fashioning forms of enslavement under the guise of "behavior control."

As I stated at the beginning of this book, the issues are not so much those of knowledge as they are of power. As things now stand, one group—scientists—have all the power. Their accountability for this power does not, as a rule, extend beyond that demanded by their professional peers. This must be changed. We cannot continue to allow respect for "expertise" and "professionalism" to blind us to the basically ideological questions that are involved in behavior control, genetic engineering, and human experimentation. They are as ideological as wage and price controls, for instance. Obviously none of us would consent to living in a country where the setting of our wage scales was left to the whims of "experts." Neither should we allow decisions that will affect the most intimate aspects of our lives be made for us by biotechnologic specialists.

The only *real* solution—the only meaningful bioethics —must start by emphasizing the basically *social* nature of biomedical technology. In a sense it is a social science. The medical and technological aspects, while they receive the most attention, are really the least important. Technical expertise can, perhaps, provide us with a clear formulation of the possibilities for, say, behavior control, but of more ultimate importance are our decisions regarding its use. We will be the ones who will somehow have to live with behavior control. Without sounding alarmist, I am convinced of the immediate importance of finding ways of stimulating widespread public involvement in these issues.

Ten years from now the decisions will have been made,

and I hope not by default, about goals and directions in bio-medical technology. Depending on our choices, we may or may not have our test-tube babies, our remote-control telemetry for "disturbed behavior," or even our "miracle cure" for cancer derived, ultimately, from the model of human experimentation we finally settle on. Looking back then, the questions challeng-ing us now will seem deceptively simple. How could we not have seen the answers all along?

All that was asked of each one of us was the courage to become involved in affirming a concept of humanity that will work for everyone.

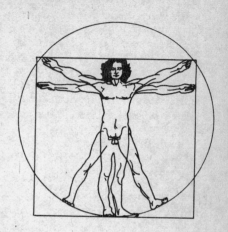

Notes
Index

Notes

Part One

Psychosurgery and the
Cult of Behavior Control

Of Chimpanzees, Ice Picks, and Madmen

3–4   The Andy quotations are from a talk at the National Institutes of Mental Health, February 1973.

4   Dr. Andy has recently been prohibited from performing psychosurgery at the University of Mississippi.

4–5   The Moniz-Fulton exchange is from a speech by Steven L. Chorover of Massachusetts Institute of Technology given at the Boston University Symposium on Psychosurgery, December 1, 1973. See also, Richard M. Restak, "The Promise and Peril of Psychosurgery," *Saturday Review–World*, September 1973, p. 54; and Steven L. Chorover, "The Pacification of the Brain," *Psychology Today*, May 1974, p. 59.

5–6   The "gold-plated icepick" information is from interviews with several neurologists and neurosurgeons in Washington, D.C.

7   The difficulty in operating on the hypothalamus is from a draft of the National Institute of Neurological Diseases and Stroke "Report on the Research Aspects of the Neurological Basis of Aggressive (Violent) Behavior," p. 11.

8   For details on tardive dyskinesia, see G. E. Crane and R. Gardner, *Psychotropic Drugs and Dysfunctions of the Basal Ganglia. A Multidisciplinary Workshop* (Washington, D.C.: Public Health Service, 1968). George Crane is a very courageous man. At a time when the drug companies enjoyed almost unlimited power to euphemize harmful drug consequences, he persisted in the unpopular truth that the major tranquilizers had serious and often irreversible consequences. Perhaps someone will eventually be able to tell the exciting story of how the truth about the major tranquilizers was finally brought to public attention, despite efforts by the drug companies to suppress this information. At the present time it has finally taken hold on the medical consciousness, and we are now reading

the same things out of Harvard and Yale that Dr. Crane was patronized for ten years ago, when his papers first appeared from Spring Grove State Hospital.

8   Interview with Ayub Ommaya, director of the research section of the National Institute of Neurologic Diseases and Stroke.

10   One notable exception to the reluctance to operate on schizophrenics is Desmond Kelley at the Atkinson Morley Hospital, London. See his "Stereotactic Limbic Leucotomy: A Preliminary Report on Forty Patients," *British Journal of Psychiatry* 123, no. 573 (August 1973): 141. Dr. Kelley's invitation to me in September 1973 to visit his ward and personally study his patients was abruptly withdrawn when he learned that my interest in psychosurgery stemmed from more than just the curiosity of a practicing neurologist.

10–11   NINDS violence study. "Aggression" is a meaningless term without reference to the social situation in which it occurs. A good summary of the current data on this can be found in NINDS, "Report on the Research Aspects of the Neurological Basis of Aggressive (Violent) Behavior," especially the section entitled "What Do Neurochemical, Endocrine, Pharmacological, and Genetic Studies Tell Us about Aggressive (Violent) Behavior?: Neurochemical and Pharmacological Studies of Aggression Using Animal Models." See also, Richard M. Restak, "Brain Pacemakers Will Watch More than the Brain," *The New York Times,* July 7, 1974.

11   For a lucid and fascinating description of the effects of brain stimulation in evoking *felt* experiences, see Wilder Penfield, *Epilepsy and the Functional Anatomy of the Human Brain* (London: J. & A. Churchill, 1954).

11–12   Many psychiatrists who have read this manuscript have been uncomfortable with the statement that temporal-lobe epileptics are indistinguishable from schizophrenics on examination. The interested reader can see for himself that this is correct. The key reference is in Eliot Slater and A. W. Beard, "The Schizophrenia-like Psychoses of Epilepsy," *British Journal of Psychiatry* 109 (1963).

12   Conversation with Murray A. Falconer, September 7, 1973, at his office at Maudesley Hospital, London.

12   For the clearest statement of Falconer's results, see "Reversibility of Temporal-Lobe Resection of the Behavioral Abnormalities of Temporal-Lobe Epilepsy," *New England Journal of Medicine* 289, no. 9 (August 30, 1973) : 451. In the same issue is an editorial by neurologist Norman Geschwind entitled "Effects of Temporal-Lobe Surgery on Behavior."

The Law and Julio Martinez
13   Data on the Millard Wright case is from George Annas, "Psychosurgery: the Law's Response" (paper presented at the Symposium on Psychosurgey, December 1, 1973, by the Center for Law and Health Sciences, Boston University Law School).

14   The Michigan case proceedings can be found in *Kaimowitz* v. *Department of Mental Health*, 2 Prison L. Rptr. 433 (August 1973), in which the opinion of the three-judge panel is set forth. Also helpful is 42 U.S.L.W. 2063 (July 31, 1973; Wayne County Circuit Court). For Smith's testimony, see Proceedings, April 4, 1973, and Post-trial Brief of Amicus Curia, American Orthopsychiatric Association, Civil Action No. 73–19434–A.W. These documents are available from the Mental Health Law Project, Washington, D.C.

15   The bill, H.R.6852, prohibits psychosurgery in federally connected health-care facilities.

15–16   Annas's remarks are from his "Psychosurgery: the Law's Response."

17   For a description of the cerebellar stimulator, see Irving Cooper and M. Riklon, *The Cerebellum, Epilepsy, and Behavior* (New York: Plenum Press, 1973). See, particularly, "The Effect of Chronic Stimulation of the Cerebellar Cortex on Epilepsy in Man" in that volume. See also, "Stimulator over Cerebellum Controls Intractable Epilepsy," *Medical Tribune*, September 5, 1973.

19–20   Riklon's work is summarized in "Psychological Studies of Chronic Cerebellar Stimulation in Man," in Cooper and Riklon, *The Cerebellum* . . .

20   The applications of cerebellar stimulation for behavior control have been carefully and sensitively discussed by Harmon L. Smith of the Divinity School, Duke University, in a paper which is reprinted in Cooper and Riklon, *The Cerebellum . . .* , "Some Ethical Considerations of Cerebellar Stimulation as an Innovative Therapy in Humans." Data were also obtained from an interview with Smith, November 15, 1973.

21   Neville's remarks are from a conversation in December 1973. A philosopher and former director of the behavior-control section at the Hastings Center, Neville has recently allied himself with psychosurgeon Vernon H. Mark. See their "Brain Surgery in Aggressive Epileptics, Social and Ethical Implications," *Journal of the American Medical Association*, no. 12 (1973) : 765. "Recently eighteen patients were committed to a mental hospital at one of our best university centers who turned out to have tumors of their limbic brains. In many cases the true nature of this illness was not recognized until the tumor had caused the patient's death." A good counterpoint providing views from the other side of the psychosurgery question can be found in almost any of the articles by the Washington psychiatrist Peter Breggin. See his "Is Psychosurgery on the Upswing?" *Human Events*, May 5, 1973. A stunning response to Dr. Breggin can be found in Henry Miller, "Psychosurgery and Dr. Breggin," *New Scientist*, July 27, 1972, p. 188.

A Way Out

21–23   Conversation with Dr. David Allen, December 6, 1973. Earlier in the month I attended a "mock" demonstration of Dr. Allen's multidisciplinary review committee.

25–26   These points were developed at the conclusion of my article "The Promise and Peril of Psychosurgery," *Saturday Review–World*, September 1973, p. 54. They still represent what I think is a sensible approach. Not surprisingly in the present climate, my name has been included among psychosurgery "advocates" and "brain mutilators" since the article's publication.

28   *Journal of the American Medical Association*, September 9, 1957, p. 695.

28–31   For background on the LEAA, see Public Law 90–351, 90th Congress, H.R.5037, June 19, 1968; and its amendment, Public Law 93–83, 93rd Congress, H.R.8152, August 6, 1973. Since I wrote this section, several reviews have appeared detailing the story of the LEAA's funding of psychosurgery and behavior modifications. See Charles Hite, "LEAA 'Clarifies' Cutoff of Behavior Mod Funds," *Psychiatric World News* 9, no. 11 (June 5, 1974); and Sharland Trotter and Jim Warren, "LEAA Drops Research Support," *Monitor* 5, no. 4 (1974).

      One of the key figures behind the investigation of the LEAA's involvement was Senator Sam Ervin. See "LEAA Halts Behavior Modification Funding," *Congressional Record*, February 19, 1974, S–1803. This contains the full text of the correspondence between Senator Ervin and LEAA acting administrator, Donald E. Santorelli. As well as I can trace it, the input for Senator Ervin's investigation came from Ms. Diane Bauer of the Children's Defense Fund and Mr. Joseph Klutz, research assistant, Subcommittee on Constitutional Rights.

30   Vernon Mark and Frank Ervin, *Violence and the Brain* (New York: Harper & Row, 1970).

30   See Dr. William Sweet's testimony at the Hearing Before a Subcommittee on the Committee on Appropriations, U.S. Senate, 92nd Congress, 2d Session, or H.R.15417, pt. 5 (1972) : 494.

The Continued Search for an
End to Violence

31   In all, six revised proposals were presented by Dr. West in response to criticism by the COPAP (Committee Opposing Psychiatric Abuse of Prisoners). In addition, these revisions were in response to a suit filed by the COPAP on July 27, 1973, which attempted to prevent the allocation of funds to the Violence Center. I have obtained copies of all six pro-

posals. The first proposal, dated September 1, 1972, contains plans for the use of psychosurgery and remote-telemetric-control techniques. The subsequent five proposals omitted any reference to such studies, as well as removing the name of Dr. Frank Ervin from the faculty list of the Violence Center.

32   A direct statement was made by Dr. Sweet linking the Boston group (the Neuroresearch Foundation) to the Violence Center. In Dr. Sweet's Senate testimony of 1972 he said, "This testimony is being presented on behalf of the Neuropsychiatric Institute of the University of California at Los Angeles under the direction of Louis Jolyon West." And later, "I am speaking today on behalf of the chief of the Neuropsychiatric Institute of the University of California at Los Angeles and his staff—Professor West." Sweet, Senate Hearings.

32   For a review of the Atascadero controversy, see "Scaring the Devil Out," *Medical World News*, October 9, 1970, p. 29; and "Inmates' Records Doctored," *ibid.*, May 5, 1972, p. 17.

33–37   Copies of the cited research projects were obtained from Ms. Diane Bauer of the Children's Defense Fund, Washington, D.C.

33   Richard Green and Joshua Golden, investigators, "The Sexually Violent Male."

34   Robert Rubin, investigator, "Chromosomal Factors and Violent Behavior." As I point out elsewhere, the association between criminality and the XYY-chromosome pattern is far from agreed upon in the scientific community. Some recognition of this disagreement was given by Dr. Rubin in his proposed study: "Reports from other countries and from the United States have been conflicting and confusing as to whether or not there is any real differential disposition toward violence in those with an extra Y chromosome."

34   Dennis Cantwell, investigator, "Violence and Minimal Brain Damage in Children."

35   Louis Jolyon West, "UCLA Proposal #1" (Los Angeles: Center for Prevention of Violence, Neuropsychiatric Institute, September 1, 1972).

35–36   Dr. West's proposed remote-monitoring techniques were dropped in the five subsequent proposals. For more on electronic-monitoring devices, see Ralph Schwitzgebel, "Electronic Innovation in the Behavioral Sciences: A Call to Responsibility," *American Psychologist*, May 1967, p. 364; Schwitzgebel, "Development and Legal Regulation of Coercive Behavior Mod Techniques with Offenders," NIMH Center for Studies of Crime and Delinquency, Chevy Chase, Maryland, February 1971 (despite its publication only four years ago, this report is virtually unobtainable now) ; Barton L. Ingraham and Gerald W. Smith, "The Use of Electronics in the Observation and Control of Human Behavior and Its Possible Use in Rehabilitation and Parole," *Issues in Criminology* 7, no. 2 (Fall 1972).

     For discussion of some of the less controversial aspects of remote telemetry applied to the brain, see Richard M. Restak, "Brain Pacemakers Would Watch More than Brain," *The New York Times,* July 7, 1974.

36   Richard Laws, investigator, "Errorless Extinction of Deviant Sexual Interest."

37   Letter from Richard Laws to Bernard Weiner, *San Francisco Chronicle.*

37–38   Coleman's remarks are from the State of California Senate Committee on Health and Welfare Hearing on Proposed Center for the Study and Reduction of Violence at UCLA, May, 1973.

38   The letter referred to is from Anthony C. Beilenson, chairman, California Legislative Senate Committee on Health and Welfare, to the author, January 8, 1974.

"Man Against Man"

39   The Edgar H. Schein article is "Man Against Man: Brainwashing," *Corrective Psychiatry and Journal of Social Therapy* 8, no. 2 (Second Quarter 1962).

40   Jessica Mitford, *Kind and Usual Punishment: The Prison Business* (New York: Alfred A. Knopf, 1973), p. 123.

40   For the description of Project START, I am indebted to Mr. Joseph Klutz, Subcommittee on Constitutional Rights, who provided copies of the START protocol.

41–42, 46–47   The Barbara Milstein quotations are from interviews in March 1974. The official position of the National Prison Project was set forth earlier this year in the "Statement of the National Prison Project on Medical Experimentation in Prisons," available from the National Prison Project, Washington.

42   Harold Cohen's comments are from his sixteen-page critique of Project START. A summary of the testimony of all the expert witnesses can be found in "Bureau of Prisons Stops START," *Psychiatric World News* 9, no. 5 (March 6, 1974).

43   The Alvin Bronstein quote is excerpted from "Federal Judge Declares Prison Behavior Modification Procedures Unconstitutional," a statement released August 2, 1974, by the National Prison Project.

43   Theodore Swift's comments are from "Bureau of Prisons Stops START" article.

43–47   Dr. Martin Groder is indeed a controversial and perplexing character. His own publications regarding Asklepieion can be found in "Asklepieion—An Effective Treatment Method for Incarcerated Character Disorders" and "Asklepieion: Effective Treatment for Felons." Both papers are reprinted as part of Groder's testimony at the Hearing Before the Subcommittee on Courts, Civil Liberties, and the Administration of Justice on Behavior Modification Programs in the Federal Bureau of Prisons, Serial no. 26, February 27, 1974. Available from the U.S. Government Printing Office, Washington, D.C.

44   The Eric Berne quotes are from *Principles of Group Treatment*.

44–45   Dr. Groder's remarks are from "Butner: Experimental U.S. Prison Holds Promise, Stirs Trepidation," *Science*, August 2, 1974, p. 423. See also Groder's statement before the House Judiciary Committee.

46   The Contingency Management Program material is from Bob Kuttner, "Virginia Prison Tests Behavior Modification," *The Washington Post*, August 11, 1974, p. B1.

46–47   For a detailed analysis of the failures of our present prison system, see David J. Rothman, "Decarcerating Prisoners and Patients," *Civil Liberties Review*, Fall 1973.

Wombs for Hire

53   The description of the *in vitro* technique is from an interview with Patrick G. Steptoe in his laboratory at Oldham General Hospital, Manchester, England, October 4, 1973.

56   The story of Frosty can be found in "Bullseye," *Nature* 243 (June 15, 1973) : 371.

56   Beatrice Mintz's work has been reported in *American Zoologist* 2 (1962) : 432; *Journal of Experimental Zoology* 157 (1964) : 273; *Proceedings of the U.S. National Academy of Science* 58 (1967) : 334, 592.

57   For data on the "zebra child," thanks are due to W. Gary Flamm, National Institute of Environmental Health Sciences, National Institutes of Health.

58   The Shope virus material is from Stanfield Rogers, "Genetic Engineering—A Potentially Invaluable Aid to Medicine and Mankind" (paper submitted to *New Scientist*).

59   Dr. Gurdon's experiments are reported in "Sexually Mature Individuals of Xenopus Laevis from the Transplantation of Single Somatic Nuclei," *Nature* (London), 182 (1958) : 64–65.

59   The McClaren mouse vertebral experiment is simply and concisely described in *Human Reproduction* (London: Granada Publishing, 1971), p. 68.

61   See "Human Births Reported from Eggs Fertilized in Lab," *The New York Times*, July 16, 1974; "First Test-Tube Babies Born," *The Washington Post*, July 16, 1974. The National Academy of Science's panel report is entitled, "Assessing Biomedical Technologies: Prospects and Problems."

61–63   The three hypothetical cases are drawn from the NAS report.

63–64   The Leon Kass material is from interviews in November 1973.

       An excellent source book for the bioethical issues raised by embryo transfer and artificial insemination is *Law and Ethics of AID and Embryo Transfer,* Ciba Foundation Symposium 17, 1973. Elsevier Excerpta Medica (North Holland: Associated Scientific Publishers).

The Genetics of Anonymity

66–73   If guidelines on sperm banking are ever drawn, it will be due in a large part to Mark S. Frankel, research associate in the Program of Policy Studies in Science and Technology of the George Washington University. Much of my material on sperm banking and the AID is from conversations with Frankel while he was preparing his report, "Public Policy Dimensions of Artificial Insemination and Human-Semen Cryobanking," Monograph No. 18 (Washington, D.C.: Program of Policy Studies in Science and Technology, George Washington University, December 1973).

66–67   The story of the seven women artificially inseminated is by Ann McClaren, "Biological Aspects of AID," in *Law and Ethics of AID and Embryo Transfer*.

67   The cattle-breeding data are from the Milk Marketing Board, "Report of the Breeding and Reproduction Organization," no. 20, 1970.

68   The quote on AID children is from Iizuka *et al.*, "The Physical and Mental Development of Children Born Following Artificial Insemination," *International Journal of Fertility* 13 (January–March 1968) : 24–32.

68   The data on the experience in the United States up to 1957 come from Schellen, *Artificial Insemination in the Human* (Amsterdam: Elsevier, 1957).

68   The figure of 10,000 birth by means of AID in 1966 is from S. J. Behrman, "Techniques of Artificial Insemination," in S. J. Behrman and R. W. Kistner, eds., *Progress in Infertility* (London: Churchill, 1968).

68–69   The data on sperm banking are from Frankel, "Artificial Insemination."

72   The Kety study can be found in S. S. Kety *et al.*, "The Types and Prevalence of Mental Illness in the Biological and Adoptive Families of Adopted Schizophrenics," *Journal of Psychiatric Research* 6 (1968, suppl. 1) : 345–62. This material was also developed during a conversation with Dr. Kety on May 3, 1974, in New York City. Much of this data is from a letter from Dr. Kety to the author, December 20, 1973.

The Third Wish

75–77   The amniocentesis material is from Fritz Fuchs, "Amniocentesis: Techniques and Complications," in Maureen Harris, ed., *Early Diagnosis of Human Genetic Defects, Scientific and Ethical Considerations* (Washington, D.C.: National Institutes of Health, 1972). Much of the same material was developed during a conversation with Dr. Cedric Carter at the Institute of Child Health, London, September 28, 1973.

76–80   The Dr. Cecil B. Jacobson material is from interviews in August 1973.

80–84   The Jack Singer quotations are from an interview at Guy's Hospital, London, September 26, 1973.

83   The reference to a girls' school offering a master's degree in genetic counseling is from the remarks of Dr. James V. Neel, Department of Human Genetics, University of Michigan Medical School, in Bruce Hilton, *et al.*, eds., *Ethical Issues in Human Genetics* (New York: Plenum, 1973).

84–85   Dr. Robert F. Murray's remarks are from "Screening: A Practitioner's View," in Hilton, Callahan, *et al.*, eds., *Ethical Issues in Human Genetics*.

85   I am indebted to Drs. Arnold Sorsley and Robert Murray for the tylosis example.

85–87   The problems associated with testicular feminization are discussed by Herbert A. Lubs, "Privacy and Genetic Information," in *Ethical Issues in Human Genetics*.

What Price the Perfect Baby?

87   The story of the divinity student is from Dr. Harmon Smith, Divinity School, Duke University, Durham, N.C.

87   The story of the mother of the mentally retarded son was described in an interview with Dr. John Fletcher of Interfaith, Washington, D.C., and of the Institute of Society, Ethics, and the Life Sciences, Hastings-on-Hudson, N.Y.

88–90   Dr. Fletcher's experimental study on the effect of amniocentesis on family structure was published as "The Bridge," *Theological Studies,* September 1972.

90–91 Dr. Kass's remarks are from interviews with the author in November 1973. Similar material was also published in "What Price the Perfect Baby?" *Science* 173 (July 9, 1971) : 103, from which the title of this section was borrowed. For an in-depth review of the whole subject of "genetic engineering," see Kass's "New Beginnings in Life," in Michael Hamilton, ed., *The New Genetics and the Future of Man* (Grand Rapids: William B. Eerdman, 1972).

Warning: Genetics May Be Hazardous to Your Health

91 The Jacobs study was first published in *Nature* 208 (1965) : 1351.

92 For a description of the technique of fluorescent staining, see "Dyeing the Y Chromosome," *Lancet,* February 6, 1971, p. 275.

92 The Hook citation is "Behavioral Implications of the Human XYY Genotype," *Science* 179 (January 12, 1973) : 139–49.

93 The sickle-cell advertisements appeared in *Ebony*, among other magazines.

93 The Arno Matulsky quotation is from "The Significance of Genetic Disease," *Ethical Issues in Human Genetics*.

94 The historical data on sickle-cell disease are from Harrison's *Principles and Practices of Internal Medicine*.

96 The Panther article appeared in an issue of *Black Panther* in 1971.

96 The TV episode is reported by Dr. Robert F. Murray, Chief of Medical Genetics at Howard University, Washington, D.C.

96 The Robinson quotation is from a letter to the author, October 1973.

96–97 An excellent article detailing the social complexities of sickle-cell research is by Tabitha M. Powledge, "The New Ghetto Hustle," *Saturday Review* 1, no. 7 (January 27, 1973).

See also, "Hazards of Indiscriminate Screening," *New England Journal of Medicine* 283 (December 31, 1970) : 1485.

97 The National Academy of Science Study is "The S-Hemoglobinopothies: An Evaluation of Their Status in the Armed Forces" (Ad Hoc Committee on S-Hemoglobinopothies, National Academy of Sciences, National Research Council, February 1973).

97 The George J. Kidera quotation is from a United Air Lines press release, March 22, 1973.

97–98 The Rodney Vessels story is from "Sickle-Cell Trait Carrier Has to Leave A.F. Academy," *The Washington Post*, July 9, 1973, p. C1.

98–100 Much of the material on the eugenics movement in the United States is from a little-known but starkly powerful book by Mark H. Haller, *Eugenics* (New Brunswick, N.J.: Rutgers University Press, 1963).

100–101 The Carrie Buck decision is recorded in *Bell* v. *Buck*, 51 ALR, 855 (1924).

Some Proposals
103 Arthur R. Jensen, "How Much Can We Boost IQ and Scholastic Achievement?" *Harvard Educational Review* 39 (1969) : 1–123; Richard J. Herrnstein, "IQ," *The Atlantic* 228 (September 1971) : 43–64.

A Game of Russian Roulette

111   The quotation on Russian roulette is from a statement by Vernon G. Cave, director, Bureau of Venereal Disease Control, Department of Health, New York City, at the Hearings of the Subcommittee on Health: *Quality of Health Care —Human Experimentation*, April 30, 1973, pt. 4. The Subcommittee hearings constitute a small text on the Tuskegee syphilis study.

111   The Charles Pollard story is from "Tuskegee Syphilis Experiment Allows 400 Alabama Black Men to Suffer without Treatment," *Ebony*, November 1972.

112   The data on mortality and morbidity are from Vernon Cave's statement, *Quality of Health Care Hearings*, p. 1234–35.

112–13   Peter Buxton was an interviewer for the Public Health Service assigned in 1966 to the Venereal Disease Clinic in San Francisco. The data on Tuskegee obtained from Buxton's investigation were presented to Ms. Heller of the Associated Press, who wrote "Syphilis Victims Went Untreated in Study," *Charlotte Observer*, July 26, 1972, p. 4A.

113–14   For a full report on Tuskegee, see "Final Report of the Tuskegee Syphilis Study Ad Hoc Advisory Panel" (Washington, D.C.: U.S. Department of Health, Education, and Welfare, Public Health Service, April 1973). See also, "Tuskegee Controversy," *Obstetrics and Gynecological News* 8, no. 19 (October 1, 1973) : 41–46.

114–15   A partial list of publications on Willowbrook includes: *Journal of the American Medical Association* 200 (1967) : 365; 212 (1970) : 1019; 218 (1971) : 1665. See also, *New England Journal of Medicine* 288 (1973) : 755. For a discussion of the issues, including a defense by Dr. Saul Krugman, see "Ethical Issues in Human Experimentation; the Case of Willowbrook State Hospital Research," published May 1972 by the Urban Health Affairs Program, New York University Medical Center, 550–560 First Avenue, New York, N.Y. 10016.

115–16   The Beecher article, probably the most influential single statement on the bioethics of human experimentation, can be found in *New England Journal of Medicine* 274 (1966) :

1354. The ideas developed in this article are given a somewhat more detailed presentation in Beecher's *Research and the Individual* (Boston: Little Brown, 1970).

116 The Ingelfinger quotation is from *Yearbook of Medicine 1967–68* (Chicago: Yearbook Medical Publishers, 1969), p. 429.

116 The *Lancet* editorial as well as the debate among its readers can be found in *Lancet* 1 (1971) : 966, 1078, and 1181; and *ibid* 2 (1971) : 95.

117 Dr. Ingelfinger's response is from a letter to the author, February 12, 1974.

What Man Has Done to Man

118–20 The Vikenti Verassayev material is from *The Memoirs of a Physician*, Simeon Linden, trans. (New York: Alfred A. Knopf, 1916), particularly pp. 332–66. I am grateful to Dr. Jay Katz of Yale University Law School for bringing this book to my attention.

121 The historical data on human experimentation are from "Historical Antecedents," in Mark S. Frankel, *The Public Health Service Guidelines Governing Research Involving Human Subjects: An Analysis of the Policy-Making Process* (Washington, D.C.: Program of Policy Studies in Science and Technology, George Washington University, February 1972). Another excellent summary is by Bradford H. Gray, *Conduct of Human Experimentation in Medical Research* (New York: John Wiley, 1975). Professor Gray was kind enough to make a prepublication copy of his book available to me during the writing of this section.

121 One of the best books on the Nazi horrors is Alexander Mitscherlich and Fred Mielke, *Doctors of Infamy: The Story of the Nazi Medical Crimes* (New York: Henry Schuman, 1949). A more philosophical examination of the same phenomena can be found in Leo Alexander, "Medical Science under Dictatorship," *New England Journal of Medicine* 241, no. 2 (July 14, 1949) : 39–47.

122–23　The Nuremberg Code is from *United States* v. *Karl Brandt et al.*, United States Adjutant General's Department, Trials of War Criminals Before Nuremberg Military Tribunals under Control Council Law No. 10 (October 1946–April 1949), the Medical Case, vol. 2 (1947).

123　　　The thirty-eight figure is from Gray, *Conduct of Human Experimentation*.

Monsters or Saints?

123–24　The Bernard Barber material is from an interview in New York City, May 2, 1974, as well as from Barber, John J. Lally, *et al.*, *Research on Human Subjects: Problems of Social Control in Medical Experimentation* (New York: Russell Sage Foundation, 1973).

125　　　The Barber-Lally experiment is described in their "The Compassionate Physician: Frequency and Social Determinants of Physician-Investigator Concern for Human Subjects," a manuscript of which was kindly provided by Dr. Barber.

126　　　The Renée Fox book is *Experiment Perilous* (Glencoe, Ill.: Free Press, 1959).

127–28　The Katz material is from an interview in January 1973 and from his *Experimentation with Human Beings* (New York: Russell Sage Foundation, 1972). This work is literally an encyclopedic compendium of readings on bioethics. It is probably the best single source book on the subject.

The Opening Wedge

131–34　The L-Dopa experiments in Huntington's chorea are published in Harold Klawans *et al.*, "Use of L-Dopa in the Detection of Presymptomatic Huntington's chorea," *New England Journal of Medicine*, June 22, 1972, pp. 1332–34.

135–37　The Marc Lappe material is from an interview at the Hastings Center, December 17, 1973.

Researchers as Double Agents?

137–38   The Laud Humphreys study is from "Tearoom Trade
—Impersonal Sex in Public Places," *Trans-Action* 15 (January 1970).

139   Stanley Milgram, *Obedience to Authority, An Experimental View* (New York: Harper & Row, 1974). See also the review of the book by Steven Marcus in *The New York Times Book Review*, January 13, 1974.

139   The Erikson quotation is from "A Comment on Disguised Observation in Sociology," *Social Problems* 366 (1967) : 367–73.

139–40   Milgram's self-evaluation of the study is from *American Psychologist* 848 (1964) : 850–52.

140   The follow-up study of the psychological aftermath of Milgram's experiments is reported in Kenneth Ring *et al.*, "Mode of Debriefing as a Factor Affecting Subjective Reaction to a Milgram-type Obedience Experiment—An Ethical Inquiry," *Representative Research in Social Psychology* 67 (1970) : 68–85.

140   The Seeman quotation is from "Deception in Psychological Research," *American Psychologist* 24 (1969) : 1025–28.

The Search for Solutions

141   The Irving Ladimer quote is from "Socio-Medico-Legal Aspects of Human Experimentation," *Journal of Public Law* 3 (1954) : 467.

141–54   The material for this section was developed from interviews with Mark Frankel, Donald Chalkley, Bernard Barber, and Jay Katz.

142   The animal kidney-transplant episode is from Frankel, *Public Health Service Guidelines*.

142–43   For the Jewish Chronic Disease Hospital case, see "Two Physicians Put on Year's Probation," *The New York Times*, December 15, 1965, p. 58; and Regents Committee on

Discipline, University of the State of New York, *Report on the Matter of Southham and Mandel*, nos. 158, 159.

143–44 Copies of all the research guidelines since 1963 can be obtained from the Institutional Relations Branch of the National Institutes of Health, 5333 West Bard Avenue, no. 303, Bethesda, Md. 20014.

144 The documents referred to are: World Medical Association, "Declaration of Helsinki" (Helsinki, Finland, 1964); Medical Research Council of Great Britain, "Responsibility in Investigations on Human Subjects," *British Medical Journal* 2 (July 18, 1964): 178–79.

145 Department of Health, Education, and Welfare, Office of the Secretary, "Protection of Human Subjects," *Federal Register* 39, no. 105 (May 30, 1974), pt. 2.

146 A comprehensive criticism of the new HEW guidelines can be found in "A Preliminary Analysis of the Draft HEW Guidelines for the Protection of Special Subjects in Biomedical Research" prepared by the staff of the Joseph and Rose Kennedy Institute for the Study of Human Reproduction and Bioethics, Georgetown University, Washington, D.C.

146–49 The Chalkley material is from an interview on January 22, 1974.

150 H.R.7724 is known as the National Research Act. Much of my discussion of the bill is from a memorandum from Mr. Joseph Klutz to Senator Sam Ervin, September 21, 1973. Similar material was also developed in conversations with Mr. Klutz in July 1974. A detailed criticism of the bill is available from the American Civil Liberties Union, Washington, D.C.

151 The National Human Investigation Board was first described in Part V of "Final Report of the Tuskegee Syphilis Study Ad Hoc Advisory Panel."

152–54 The Capron material was from an interview at the University of Pennsylvania Law School, April 25, 1974. See also, Capron's "Legal Considerations Affecting Clinical Pharmacological Studies in Children," *Clinical Research* 21 (1972). Also, "Protection of Human Subjects," *Science*, March 1, 1974, p. 797.

157–61 The material on the council is from interviews with Jerome K. Ravetz in London during September–October 1973. For the initial statement of council aims, see Paul Sieghart, "Science and Social Ethics: A Corporate Conscience for the Scientific Community?" *Nature* 239, no. 5366 (September 1, 1972) : 15–18. See also, Nicholas Wade, "Science and Society: British Group to Be Harbinger of Dangers," *Science* 181 (August 3, 1973) : 420–21.

161–62 The Steven Rose quotations are from an interview at his home in London, September 26, 1973. Quotations are also taken from Hilary Rose and Steven Rose, *Science and Society* (Baltimore, Md.: Penguin Books, 1969).

Index

Abortion, debate over, xv, 169; in embryo transfer, 55; and embryo-transfer discards, 65; and genetic counseling, 82, 88, 105; and mongolism, 77–78; protections of fetus in, 145, 153; and sex-linked diseases, 80

Aggression, alleged neuropathology of, 3, 28, 30, 47; and androgen metabolism, 33; chromosomal abnormality and, 34, 91–93; in epilepsy, 11–12, 17–20; and minimal brain dysfunction, 34–35; predatory as opposed to shock-induced, 10–11; psychosurgery for, 3, 10–11; tranquilizers and, 11; *see also* Violence

Alcoholism, 35, 70, 71, 98, 99

Allen, David F., 21–24

Almeida Lima, 5

American Civil Liberties Union (ACLU), 41, 43, 45–46

Amniocentesis (prenatal diagnosis), complications of, 76–77; errors in, 83–84; and genetic disease, 75–78, 87–89; and genetic "silent carriers," 79–80; history of, 61, 75; and preselection, 78, 88; recent advances in, 81–82; technique of, 76

Amygdalotomy, 8, 33n

Androgens, 33

Andy, Orlando J., 3–4, 48

Annas, George J., 15–16, 25, 27

Anthropometry, 98

Antibiotics, xiv, 58, 112–13, 159

Antidepressant drugs, xiv, 160

Arginine, 57–58

Armed Forces Epidemiologic Board, 114

Artificial insemination, applications of, 66, 68–69; of cattle, 67; and deep-frozen technique, 68–69; history of, 67–68; technique of, 67

Artificial insemination by donors (AID), 67–73, 103; compared with blood donation, 70–71; and genetic inheritance, xvi, 70–73, 104; secrecy of, 67, 69; and sperm banks, 69–71

Artificial organs, 131

Asklepieion Society, 45

Astronomy, as Babylonian technology, 162

Atomic bomb, 106, 131, 140

"Attack therapy" (Asklepieion therapy), 38, 40, 43–45

"Bad genes," 79, 88–89

"Bad seed," 98

"Balanced carrier," 83–84

Barber, Bernard, 123–27, 151

Barr, Dr., 100

Beaumont, William, 121

Becky (chimpanzee), 4

Beecher, Henry K., 116

Behavior modification, 3–50; as behavior "control," xi, xvi, 47–50; and constitutional rights of prisoners, 13–15, 41–43; by indoctrination, 32n–33n, 39–47; of institutionalized subjects, xii, xvi, 13–15, 32, 32n–

33n, 35–47, 167; in penal "treatment" programs, xvi, 32n–33n, 40–47, 169; political implications of, xii, 25, 27–50, 169; and prison system, 46–47; psychiatric approaches to, 31–47; and surgery, 3–27; therapies for, 32, 32n–33n, 36–37, 39–47; and U.S. government support, xvi, 27–30, 32, 36–43, 46, 47; *see also* Psychosurgery

"Behavioral Implications of the Human XYY Genotype," 92

"Behavioral instrumentation," 36

Bell, J. H., 101

Bennett, James V., 39

Berne, Eric, 44

Berstein, Sharon and Terry, 73–74

Bevis, Douglas, 61

Bicknell, Ernest, 99

Bioethics, *passim*; formulation of, xii–xiii, 141–70; imperative of, 49

Biofeedback, 25

"Biological Predicters in Early Childhood of Subsequent Impaired Impulse Control" (study proposal), 36

Biomedical research, and the individual patient, 118, 126–28; and law enforcement, 27–32, 32n–33n, 36–38; predictive, 30, 31–32, 34–36, 54–56, 75–87, 91–93, 96–97, 131, 134–37; and social solutions, 11, 47–49, 104–105, 115, 161–62; U.S. government funding of, xiii, xvi, 27–31, 32, 36–38, 47, 49, 111, 113, 142–43, 145–46, 150; *see also* Biomedical technology, Genetic screening, Medical researchers, Pretesting

Biomedical technology, of applied genetics, 53–107; as autonomous "state," 130; democratization of, 161–62; elitism of, xiii, 23, 73, 103, 106, 130, 161–162, 169; and ethical absolutes, xii–xiii, 78; in human experimentation, 111–36, 141–64; as ideology, 169; imminence of, xiv; and limits of power, xii–xiii, 66, 73, 82, 106, 117, 130, 135–36, 143, 161–62, 168–69; mythic neutrality of, 162–63; as "prostitute," 158–59; of psychosurgery and behavior modification, 3–38, 47–50; and public debate, xv, 27, 49, 102, 106–107, 157, 159–63, 168–69; and race, 93–98, 101–102, 103, 111–13, 145; and response time to consequences, xiv–xv, 156–157; as social control, 25, 27–38, 47–50, 78, 90–92, 97–107, 135–36, 162–63, 169; social revolution of, xi; and societal responsibility, xviii, 23–27, 49–50, 73, 102–107, 130–31, 154–162, 168–70; *see also* Psychiatry, Social science

"Blighted ova," 83

Blood donors, 70

Bockhart, Max, 119

Bowman, James F., 97

Brainwashing, 38–43

British Society for Social Responsibility in Science (BSSRS), 157, 161

Bronstein, Alvin J., 43

Brown, Bertram, 19

Buck, Carrie, 100–101

Buck v. *Bell*, 100–101

Bunn, Ernest, 119

Bureau of Prisons, 39–40, 42–43, 46, 144, 146, 150

Buxton, Peter, 112

California Council for Criminal Justice (CCCJ), 32, 37
Cancer, 85, 86, 143, 168
Capron, Alexander, 151–54
Carrier states (of recessive genes), 79–80, 84–85, 104; and sickle-cell trait, 93–98
Castration, of the feebleminded, 99–100
Cave, Vernon G., 111
Center for the Prevention of Violence, 31–33, 35, 37–38, 48
Cerebellar electrical stimulator, 17; distinguished from psychosurgery, 19–20; legal status of, 20–21; technique of, 18–19
Cerebellum, 18–19
Chalkley, Donald, 146–49
Chimera, 56–57
Chorea, 132–33; see also Huntington's chorea
"Chromosomal Factors and Violent Behavior" (study proposal), 34–35
Chromosomes, abnormalities of, 34, 54, 70, 77, 80–81, 84, 91–92; and criminality, 34, 91–93, 98, 101; genes of, 74–75, 79, 103, 104; in mongolism and other genetic diseases, 74–77; and sex-linked diseases, 56, 79–80; techniques for study of (embryo transfer, amniocentesis), 54, 74–75; in testicular feminization, 86; translocation of, 74–75, 81
Cingulotomy, 8
Clark, Robert, 97
Cohen, Harold, 42
Coleman, Lee, 37–38
"Comment on Disguised Observation in Sociology, A," 139

Committee Opposing Psychiatric Abuse of Prisoners (COPAP), 37–38
Committee to Evaluate START, 42
Computer, behavioral monitoring by, 36; data banks, xii, 156
Conscious Brain, The, 161
Contingency Management Program (CMP), 46
Cooper, Irving, 17–20
Corrective Psychiatry and Journal of Social Therapy, 39
Council for Science and Society, The, xviii, 157–63, 168
Criminology, 98
Curran, William J., 142
Cyproterone acetate, 33

Declaration of Helsinki, 144
Deep freezing (of sperm), 66; history of, 68; and infertility, 68; and "sperm market," 69; and vasectomy, 69; see also Sperm banks
Depth electrode techniques, 11, 16
Development and Legal Regulation of Coercive Behavior Mod Techniques with Offenders, 36
Diggs, Lemuel W., 94
Dow, Robert S., 18–19
Drug addiction, 43, 70, 71
Drug Amendment Act, 142
Durst (boy), 119

Eaton, David, 95
Edwards, Robert G., 53–55, 57, 59–60, 65
Eichmann, K. A., 139
Electronic surveillance, 35–36, 170
Embryo transfer, 53–66, 73, 103; and "adopted" embryo, 62; benefits of, 54–56; with celi-

Good Samaritan Medical Center, 18

Groder, Martin, 40n, 43–46

Gurdon, J. B., 59

Hallucinogenic drugs, 130

Health, Education and Welfare, Department of, 113, 141, 144–146, 150

Heart transplants, xiii, 159

Heller, Jean, 112

Hemophilia, 56, 79–80

Hepatitis, and commercial blood, 70; in Willowbrook study, 114–117

Herrick, J. B., 94

Herrnstein, Richard, 103

Heterozygotes (genetic "carriers"), 79–80

Holmes, Justice Oliver Wendell, 100–101

Homosexuality, 137–38, 139

Homozygotes, 79

Hook, Ernest, 92

Hospitals (*see also* Universities)
    Atascadero State, 32, 32n–33n, 48
    Boston City, 21, 28
    Carstairs Maximum Security, 91
    Guy's, xvi, 80, 83, 84
    Ionia State, 14–15
    Jewish Chronic Disease, 143
    Johns Hopkins, 146–47
    Massachusetts General, 28
    Maudesley, 12
    Oldham General, 60
    St. Barnabas, 17, 19
    St. Christopher's, 83
    St. Elizabeths, 6
    Vacaville, 33n

Howard, Thomas, 46

Human experimentation, 111–64, 168–70; and character of researchers, xvii, 115, 117–21, 123–28, 130, 137–38; on children, 114–17, 119–20, 153–54, 168; and community attitudes, 145–47; and "compassion" of investigators, 125–27; compensation for, 150; and concept of "harm," 138–39; ethics of, xvi–xvii, 107, 112–14, 116–17, 120–122, 124–27, 130, 135–36, 138–143, 146, 150, 154–60; HEW (NIH) guidelines for, 141–46; and individual's right to privacy, 138–41; during National Socialism, 121; preventive as opposed to punitive laws for, 148; and principles of Nuremberg Code, 122–23; and professional reputation, 159; ratio of risk to benefit in, 122–25, 143–146, 148–49, 152, 160; regulation of, xi–xii, 127–28, 131, 136, 141–64, 168–69; scandals of, 142–43; like shamanism, 135; in social sciences, xvii, 137–41; of Stanley Milgram, 139–40; subjects in, xvii, 111–121, 124, 137–39, 140–41, 151; wisdom as opposed to knowledge in, 140

Humphreys, Laud, 137–40

Hunter, John, 67

Huntington's chorea, 131–36; as affording the "opening wedge," 135

Hyperkinetic children (hyperactive children), 4, 34–35, 48–49

Hyperresponsive Syndrome, 3

In vitro fertilization, xiii, 53, 61–62, 64, 106, 167; *see also* Embryo transfer

Infertility (sterility), of men, 68–69; in women, 54, 60, 66

"Informed consent," with cerebellar-stimulation techniques,

20; and children, 145, 153–54, 168; difficulties of, xvii, 16; 128, 142, 147; in England, 144; and genetic research, 106; and the involuntarily confined, 14–15, 26, 33n, 45, 144–45; NIH definition of, 143–44; rules for, 129, 143–44, 151; of society, 130; and volunteers in hallucinogen study, 130

Ingelfinger, Franz, 116–17

Institute for Behavioral Research, 42

Institute for Cancer Research, 56

Institute of Society, Ethics, and the Life Sciences (Hastings Center), 87, 135

Institutional Human Investigation Committees (IHIC), 152

International Journal of Fertility, 68

IQ theory, 103

Jacobs, Patricia, 91–92

Jacobson, Cecil B., 77–80

Jensen, Arthur, 103

Journal of the American Medical Association, 28, 115, 116, 124–125

Justice, Department of, 28–29, 40, 45

Kansas State Home for the Feebleminded, 99

Karolinska Institute, 92

Kass, Leon, 63–65, 90

Katz, Jay, 127–31, 138, 151, 154

Kennedy, Senator Edward, 150

Kennedy bill (H.R. 7724), xviii, 150–51, 154

Kennedy Institute for the Study of Human Reproduction and Bioethics, 63

Kety, Seymour, 72

Kidera, George J., 97

Kind and Usual Punishment, 40

Klawans, Harold, 134

Krugman, Saul, 116

Ladimer, Irving, 141

Lally, John J., 125

Lancet, 116

Langley-Porter Neuropsychiatric Institute, 43–44

Lappe, Marc, xvii, 135–37

Law Enforcement Assistance Administration (LEAA), 28–30, 32, 46, 48, 146

Laws, Richard, 37

L-Dopa, 9; and detection of Huntington's chorea, 134–35

Lead poisoning, 104–105

Lehman, Herman, 94

Leukemia, 92, 168

Limbic encephalitis, 10

Limbic system, 6–10

Lombroso, Cesare, 98

Lowell, Josephine Shaw, 99

Lubs, Herbert, 96

Lucy (chimpanzee), 4

"Man Against Man," 39

Mandel, Emanuel E., 142–43

Manhattan Project, 106

Mantegazza, Paolo, 68

"Marijuana Use in Violent Behavior" (study proposal), 36

Mark, Vernon, 16, 21–24, 28, 30, 32, 47

Marshall, John, 129

Martinez, Julio, 17–20

Massachusetts Institute of Technology, 39

Mather, Cotton, 133

McLaren, Ann, 59, 63

Medical Committee for Human Rights, 14

Medical Registry, 72

Medical Research Council of Great Britain, 144

Medical researchers, contrasted with practicing physicians, 117–18; dehumanization of, 130; Nazi, 121; role conflict of, 126–27; like shamans, 135–36; social obligations of, 154–56; as special-interest group, 23, 163; study of, 118–20, 123–27; *see also* Biomedical research, Social science

Memoirs of a Physician, The, 118

Mentally disordered sex offenders (MDSO), 36–37

Milgram, Stanley, 139–40

Milstein, Barbara, 41–42, 45–46

Minimal-brain-damage syndrome, 34–35

Mintz, Beatrice, 56–57

Mitford, Jessica, 40

Mongolism (Down's syndrome), 54–55, 74–78, 87, 88

Moniz, Antonio Egas, 4–5

Motulsky, Arno, 93–94

Multidisciplinary review committees, xvi, 21–25, 113–14, 127, 130, 145, 147, 150, 158–59; argument against, 149; province of, 151

Multiple sclerosis, 136

Mumps, 68

Murray, Robert, 84–85

National Academy of Sciences, 58, 61, 63, 97

National Commission for the Protection of Human Subjects of Biomedical Research, 150–151

National Communicable Disease Center, 70, 112

National Distillers, Inc., xv

National Human Investigation Board (NHIB), xviii, 151–53

National Institute of Mental Health (NIMH), 13, 19, 36

National Institutes of Health (NIH), 29, 30, 141–43, 146

National Law Center, 14

National Prison Project, 41, 43, 45

National Research Council, 97

Nature, 157

Neuro Research Foundation, 28, 30, 32

Neville, Robert, 21, 26

New England Journal of Medicine, 12, 115, 116, 134

Nuclear cloning, xii, 58–60, 105, 160

Nuclear fission, xiv

Nuremberg Code, 121–23

Oak Ridge National Laboratory, 25, 58

Obedience to Authority, 139

Oliver, John W., 43

Omnibus Crime Control and Safe Streets Act, 29

Opton, Ed, 37

Oral contraceptives, xiv–xv, 147, 156

Organ transplantation, xiii, xiv, 129, 131, 142, 159

Papez, J., 6

Parkinson's disease, 9, 134

Participant observation, 137–41

Peer review, 29–30, 143, 151

Penicillin, 112, 113

"Physical and Mental Development of Children Born Following Artificial Insemination," 68

Pilcher, F. Hoyt, 99, 101

Pollard, Charles Wesley, 111–12, 115

Pollution, xiv, 160, 161

Population Council, 147

Prefrontal lobotomy (leucotomy), 5–6, 9–10